GARY R
POEMS

BY GARY MICHAEL RUDDICK

'One million people commit suicide every year.'
The World Health Organization

Gary Michael Ruddick

Published by
Chipmunkapublishing
PO Box 6872
Brentwood
Essex CM13 1ZT
United Kingdom

http://www.chipmunkapublishing.co.uk

Cover Image Nick Chapman

GARY RUDDICK POEMS

A FAREWELL IN THE FORM OF A WREATH

Alas, I was far cleverer than just your common
little thief.
In times long ago now forgotten I wore a blade of
the finest steel – sharper than an eagle's claw. For
where I learnt about life you had to be conditioned
and prepared for unpredicted grief.
Trouble was kept in the underground – dealt with
secretly, unknown to the police.
For to make that fatal mistake was something the
elders disapproved of, so we learnt young those
were our beliefs,
Most, if not all, only participated in the using of
narcotics, since it was a deeper form of spiritual
release.
There, Babylon interfered and removed those
suspected of defacing the human race and
undercover of darkness buried, those in the
corners of every cemetery for most of them are on
a government lease.
SO our memories shall never fade with the
passage of time, for those that left us lost their
lives and the fight and now are deceased,
Strange, for at this moment in time there are now
more narcotics floating on our countries streets,
The war continuous on for there is more and more
deaths and if you have insight, you will watch
them increase.

I always in my younger days believed that they were for love, harmony and peace,

I wonder if it is now political that the majority of the world is in grief,

For segments of our governments are more than just peace, now most of the countries are armed secret police,

The king of the African jungles no longer remembered as their great predator who ruled as their wild beast,

Will the hunt for the royal blue blooded most sort after fox eventually cease?

Or do those that think that they are noble once again let their hounds be released?

Just to rip and gorge on young cub that was not even a morsel, let alone a feast,

Not even old enough to defend herself with her own teeth,

For those beautiful and elegant creatures for your dead, I lay a loving tribute in the form of a wreath,

Where I scream in my soul silently yet ear piercingly sour great long lost Indian warrior who was once our chief,

His woman was in form a beautiful goddess of such power that he named her his sorcerer – for the night's mischief.

For it was his strength and wisdom that kept them for so long without war and for that she was at peace,

GARY RUDDICK POEMS

Each morning at sunrise, she would ritually prepare with skill the ancient ancestors' pipe of peace,
To stem the flow of rain that always came from the skies from the Far East,
She always foretold her chief that soon it would be time to hunt the wild buffalo beast,
For the time had once again returned for their sacred ceremonious feast. Together they smoked in silence and harmony praying to their fore fathers and their much beloved mothers who had spiritually levitated and with the fires of their passing were released into the wind, taking them through the rough planes towards the east,
The light skinned man had invaded their holy grind and stolen and slaughtered their cattle for their beef,
M any a warrior now lay silent, buried in the holy land, yet they shall never be at rest for their spirits continue to enrage the west for the land mourns her warriors crest,
The marking of the gods inscribed with colours upon his chest, for as a young brave he achieved every endurance test,
The days of yesterday still loom in the skies dark and foreboding with unrest,
Death to them is the only way that they feel their only races can now be blessed,
FOR centuries their people have been put to the test,

Stirring mysteriously in the cloud of smoke from
their fires' covers the skies with a silent yet unrest,
For too long have they lived in poverty and now
they are lost, broken, desolate and in disbelief,
Even those that have to as of yet been born are
tortured and tormented for there are those who
have the vision and they have foretold there will
be more than spiritual unease,
For man has crossed the seven seas and brought
with him disease,
Nations will one day be brought down to their
knees,
The heavens will pay attention to their pleas,
The rains shall hail down across the lands and the
Earth will forever more freeze,
For those races, fortunate to survive shall to fight
with all of their lives,
For on the warpath are those that have been,
since time began, told lies,
The wizards and sorcerers will change all their
dies,
B ringing with them the power of light from the
skies,
For they have lain in wait with silent minds and
closed eyes,
They have remembered all of those that have
died,
The heavens shall no longer be denied,
The tribes of the land came down from the sacred
mountains shall come out of hiding to survive,

GARY RUDDICK POEMS

Yet those that are allegedly now civilized will clash
and collide,
For Mother Nature for far too long has been
defied,
Because no race or religion has stood side by
side,
There fore life on earth has long ago died,
For even the groom and the bride,
Long before their vows were tied,
Promises were broken and tears were cried,
Therefore, the elements are the powers left to
decide,
The shaman a warrior of his time full of wisdom
and incantations shall one day prepare holy rituals
that only the light of the full moon shall witness.
For only he has the potion in which he can change
the direction of each and every nation,
Believe me: there shall be no intervention,
Not from all of the world's professions
For it is long gone past the date of confession,
At the end, there shall be no lost love, not even a
blessing,
The smoke signals shall never stop calling on the
warriors of all times,
The bones of the buffalo will be placed in all the
world's directions,
The elements shall find their way through the
endless years of pollution,
For there are no longer any more natural
solutions,
The chiefs from the forgotten time

Will for one last time join together in the bond that
has existed since the beginning of time
Steadied the axles and kept the world in line,
Some day their movement will cease,
The Indians put all of history together piece by
piece,
For the fires of the earth's life has all but ceased,
Which nation, race, or religion shall be the first to
be deceased?
Will every bird that has flown through the heavens,
I wonder, produce a feather of the highest
pedigree to make a magical wreath?
In honour of the world's greatest legendry chief,
Who is none other that JESUS, who was much
more than a high priest?
No longer is his spirit as one for he no longer rests
in peace,
For there are those whose souls were never
meant to be released,
The darkness that in man has increased,
For the lambs have all been fleeced,
Yet the shepherd has all paths of humankind
traced,
For on his hands are the lines of the human race,
For it is he who has that last magical illus ional
beautiful ace,
So put another star in the constellations of the
galaxy of space,
For you should always look into a person's eyes –
never the face.
Or are you one of those that's in disgrace,

GARY RUDDICK POEMS

For the likes of you can never find a hiding place.
For in our race there is no place for a racist's face,
You always speak in the worst possible taste,
The likes of you belong with the rubbish waste,
In addition, those that are labelled in the textbook as a convicted sex case,
PLEASE remove yourself from our human race,
For a long time ago you fell from grace,
So go to that hole in the ground – hurry, with haste!
For we no longer wish to see your face,
For this moment in the present time, ill rest my forensic case,
As I need to cleanse myself of this god forsaken place,
Now I shall, from this earth, my steps erase,
In addition, retire to my resting place,
Where I KNEW I should have stayed in my peaceful resting place,
I'm bowing out with me, I hope with some sort of grace,
As here I feel in a manner of speaking out of place,
For you do not know their name or their case, and you have no idea what hides behind their face,
YOU KNOW THAT FOR SURE AND YOU HAVE TO BE SURE, for they will try to invade your space,
You could, heaven forbid, become another rape or child abuse case,

IF I could, I would take your place to remove the torment you must have faced.

What have they done to our human race?

What am I doing in such a cold and dark place?

THIS really is a living hell and all I see is this decrepit face,

Now these legally labelled me as that Indian CRAZY ACE.

GARY RUDDICK POEMS

A MOTHER TO BE

My Dear friend Jane, shortly there shall be yet
another young kin to join your family tree ~$ce I
was a soldier.doc,

A further continuation of your families' bloodline
and your past, present, and future families' history,

In motherhood, I do assume that you already have
more than an honours degree,

In childbirth, there are only two courses of fertility
in which child will turn out to be,

That, therefore, is whether your baby shall be a he
or a she,

In times of old, they would have been referred to
as thee,

The process of childbirth for quite a long period of
time has captivated me,

For those who have come of age, most have
experienced those precious moments shared in
intimacy,

For those emotions and desires and love are
joined together physically and deeper still,
spiritually,

Where through the process of nature, male and
female cautions entwine as we,

In my mind's eye, when a woman reaches the
stages of pregnancy,

Therefore, through the passage of time the
woman becomes her spouse's queen bee,

So in reality they are committed to their offspring
for all of eternity,

Through are learning's of those gone before us respectfully and those that are inclined and guided religiously,

Through their studies of biology sociology psychology psychiatry or even deeper as a whole holistically,

The birth of your baby shall be noted for forever and a day,

As you will already have thought the first stages of life is acceptance,

Through my personal knowledge the bond between mother and child should always be guided patiently and lovingly,

In return, your child shall love you unconditionally,

Who knows, one day your Child's future may lie in the skies with the stars, the planets and the signs of astrology,

Where, allegedly, through our ancestors have for generations believed our ancestors and mothers are expected to be,

Therefore, educationally, your child should learn firstly their a b and c and if I can recall their one two and threes,

So those therefore are the stages of numerology,

Then there are the stages of further learning of history,

If they choose to travel further the path of geography,

Maybe the mind will allow those to open their senses to the world musically,

GARY RUDDICK POEMS

Where according to our books through history allegedly somewhere above heaven is meant to be,
Maybe someday we might be fortunate and be allowed to venture through space and time where we could live as one spiritually,
Yet some things will only progress gradually,
In the months gone by and in the forth-coming months you and your child will reach the peak of purity,
I hope that you and your baby shall retain a high level of normality,
In this world of unrest and in some respects insanity,
Who knows, maybe one day when I return to society?
In passing, we may exchange greetings socially,
However, for the time being, I hope you enjoy the time off with your maternity,
In addition, I hope that the rest of your pregnancy you can enjoy comfortably,
I hope that the arrival of your child shall arrive pleasantly,
Now is the time for myself to bow out gracefully,
Thank you for your time and your hospitality,
Warmest regards as a father respectfully and honourable,

Yours affectionately and sincerely,

A WITCHES' GATHERING

WELCOME TO THE MAGIC CIRCLE OF THE
FIRE,
WHERE EVERY WITCH OFFERS HERSELF TO
THE DEVIL FOR HIS DESIRE,
FOR IN THE REALM OF DARKNESS HE IS THE
MESSIAH,
UNDER THE PROTECTION OF THE WITCHES
HE GOES BY HIS TITLE THAT OF THE LORD,
SIRE,

PRIESTS AND PRIESTESSES WEAR THEIR
CEREMONIAL GOWNS,
HIGH PRIESTESSES WEAR THEIR GLORIOUS
CROWNS,
DRESSES MADE OF WONDERFUL COLOURS
OF SILK SATIN AND LACE,
FOR EVERY GODDESS HAS HER RIGHTFUL
PLACE,

EVERY WITCH WEARS A COVE OF GARLIC,
FOR THEIR LORD WITH HIS DEVILRY IN HIS
SOUL KNOWS EVERY TRICK,
EVERY ANGEL HAS TO ARRIVE BEFORE THE
MIDNIGHT ON HER BROOM STICK,
WATCHING THE FULL MOON HIS MIND
SECRETLY BEGINS TO CLICK,

SHADOWS FLY BY HIM FROM LEFT TO RIGHT,

GARY RUDDICK POEMS

HE DOESN'T MISS A FLICKER FOR HIS SIGHT
IS THAT OF AN OWL AT NIGHT,
FIRES AND LANTERNS HAVE NOW BEEN
ALIGHTED,
WITCHES OF ALL NATIONS ARE FOR ONCE
BEEN UNITED,

RUNES, STONES, HAVE ALL BEEN PLACED
AROUND THE FIRE,
THE DEVIL STANDS AMONGST THE FLAMES;
THEY DO NOT HARM HIM FOR THEY GROW
EVEN HIGHER,
STANDING THERE IN HIS ROYAL PURPLE AND
GOLDEN ATTIRE,
SEEKING OUT A GODDESS THAT WOULD,
FOR TONIGHT, QUENCH HIS ANIMAL DESIRE,

WITH HIS MAGIC IN FULL FLOW, HE SENSES
A GODDESS WHO IS OF ROYAL BLOOD,
WHO IS WILLING TO OFFER HIM ANOTHER
CROWN THAT WITH OWE WOULD MAKE HIM
RULER OF HER SISTERHOOD,
RAISING HIS HANDS SILENCE BEFALLS
ACROSS THE LAND,
ALONE IN THE GLIMMERING LIGHT OF THE
MOON A WOMAN DOES STAND,

THE WIND BRINGS TO HIM A SWEET
LAVENDER HEAVENLY SCENT,
KNEELING GENTLY BEFORE HIM THE WOMAN
ASKED HIM: OH WAS SHE SENT?

JOINING HER ON HIS KNEES, TAKING HER HANDS IN HIS, HE RELIED ALL MAN AND WOMAN MUST NOW REPENT,
FOR HE WAS THE FALLEN ANGEL, TO EARTH WAS WHY HE WAS REALLY SENT,

HE ASKED HER IF SHE WOULD JOIN HIM IN THE FIRE, FOR IN THE ELEMENTS THERE WAS NO HIGHER,
FOR HE HAD FALLEN IN LOVE AND THIS WAS NOT JUST ABOUT DESIRE,
THIS WAS HER DESTINY FOR HE WANTED TO BE HER CHILD'S SIRE,

WITH THAT HE STOOD AND OFFERED HER HIS HAND,
GENTLY SHE TOOK IT AND TOGETHER THEY DID STAND,
SOMETHING FLOWED THROUGH THEM AND SHE LOOKED UPON HER LEFT HAND,
UPON HER WEDDING FINGER WAS A GLEAMING FIRE STONE IN A GOLD BAND,

HE GENTLY RAISED IT TO HIS MOUTH, SPEAKING THESE WORDS TOGETHER WE SHALL FOREVER RULE THE NORTH, EAST, WEST AND SOUTH,
MAY ALL THOSE THAT FOLLOW US AND JOIN WITH US LIVE LONG AND I PRAY FOREVER STAY IN GOOD HEALTH,

GARY RUDDICK POEMS

ARMS ENTWINED WITHIN EACH OTHER, THE
RITUAL OF THE BONDING WAS ABOUT TO
BEGIN,
WHERE THOSE IN THEIR COVEN WERE NOT
ALLOWED TO SIN,

A THREAD OF GOLDEN AND SILVER SILK
WAS ENTWINED AROUND THEIR WRISTS,
ON THEIR HEADS A CROWN MADE OF ALL
GEMS; THE BIGGEST IN THE CENTRE – THE
AMETHYST,
WITH THESE WORDS HE SAID: SPIRITUALLY
YOU SHALL COME AND GO IN THE MORNING
MIST,
FOR MY HOME IS THE HEAVENS AND YOU
ARE THE HOSTESS AND NO LONGER A
GUEST,

OUT OF NOWHERE HE PRODUCED A
CRYSTAL CUP,
RAISING IT TO HER LIPS HE SAID ONLY TAKE
A SUP,
WITH THAT IN HIS ARMS HE GENTLY PICKED
HER UP,
WALKING INTO THE FIRE THE HEAVENS ALL
LIT UP,

THE MUSIC SEEMED TO COME FROM THE
SKIES,

LITTLE DID THE WITCHES KNOW HE WAS NOT
THE DEVIL FOR HE WAS THEIR HEAVENLY
LORD IN DISGUISE,
A PATHWAY IN THE STARS OPENED UP IN
THE NIGHT SKY,
WITH THE LORD AND HIS QUEEN THANKED
EVERYONE AND SAID THEIR GOODBYES.

A MAGIC SPELL HAD, BY HIS LORDSHIP AND
HIS QUEEN, BEEN CAST OVER THE
CHILDREN ALL ACROSS THE LAND,
THAT EVERY CHILD WHO WALKED THE
EARTH WOULD, ONE DAY, REACH THE
PROMISED LAND,
THEY KNEW THAT IT WOULD NOT HAPPEN
OVER NIGHT AND MANY WOULD NOT
UNDERSTAND,
FOR EVERY ONE'S DESTINY IS ENGRAVED
UPON THE LORD'S HAND.

****

And for the foreseeable future I shall have to
endure taking some form of light sedation,
So if you see me writing please do not worry about
me too much, as it's just me being my self, trying
to relieve my agitation,
In my mind I feel that I have an obligation both to
myself and those around me.
For it is so easy for someone to be imprisoned for
a wrong allegation,

GARY RUDDICK POEMS

Many incidents occur because of lack of insight and provocation,
And once again you're being accused of using violent aggression,
So therefore you're placed in a different location,
And they inject you with a mind numbing medication,
Therefore the next stage is you're diagnosed as suffering from depression,
And for days, weeks, months… you find yourself locked up in isolation,
Many a night I have peered through the bars in the hole in the wall wondering if there was any body out there to help me up there in far off constellation,
Maybe a lonesome ship wandering through space and time from a secret federation,
Alone and lost I shed a lonesome tear for I have no voice, therefore I don't have any longer any form of culmination,
The sad thing is, those that were close to me had once voiced their expectations,
I never gave it a thought to join the congregation,
I spent too much time thinking about a bail application,
Looking at the ladies in the magazines with nothing but love and adoration,
If you're old enough and unfortunate to be single you don't have much choice but to learn about self-masturbation,

For the first time it is more than a mind-blowing and physical sensation,
So you must bear with me when I argue about the effects of my medication,
And therefore, when a man can no longer get an erection,
He no longer catches the woman's attention,
I thought it was the condom that stopped you from getting an infection,
So you must understand my feeling dejection,
All I was praying for was a baby girl, yet your pills caused the prevention,
Now I'm back to the same old feeling: rejection,
And in putting my thoughts where every one can see them no longer gives me any satisfaction,
So if you think that I owe you some form of gratification,
What for? A better quality of life? I wouldn't be surprised if all of the learning concerning the mind were just a bloody fabrication,
And to top this saga off you've now induced in constipation,
And I've suddenly got this realization,
That half of you haven't a clue what you're doing as you spend most of you shift watching that damned television,
And you're all fixated by its false illusion,
I can't wait until the next revolution,
I just hope I'm not here for the mighty explosion,
It shan't be long before you all make another new year's resolution,

GARY RUDDICK POEMS

Myself, I'll just kiss my crucifixion.
For I can see us all heading for extinction,
As the saying goes that my friend is evolution.

ANOTHER SEASON

Why does any form of death has to have a reason,
It could be that it was just a change in the season,
Left alone old and frail desolate and freezing,
Are then the heavens guilty of humanitarian treason?

For are we not all the same male and female cousins,
Therefore is the money worth more than a life that you get for your political extortions,
Who will be the country to fall under the western-armed coalition?
Will thoraces and the religions all endeavour in long awaited worldwide mission,
I wonder if there are those that are silently wishing,
That they could return to their long lost youth to their innocence and petty kissing,
No one fully understands what they once had until it's lost and forever missing,
Strange don't you think? How tomorrow always keeps us guessing,
Isn't it about time that it was in our children that we started investing?
Not their minds that for so long radio and the television have been infesting,
Surely each and every child needs love and guidance and at some stage a blessing,

GARY RUDDICK POEMS

Why does every baby need to continue to physically and psychologically need more and more testing?
Why does the mind forever need continuous resting?
Is it that reality has brought about something that is dark dangerous and is somewhere unbeknown to us manifesting,
How much longer shall it be before the human races are seriously taught a worldwide lesson?
For surely that is not our idea of unity and progression,
As in my mind that a backward step isn't that regression,
Which country next shall fall and give in under submission,
FOR no dictator has ever made a confession,
Who will be the next leader to ask the waiting question?
How many more shall die from war disease and malnutrition.

ARE YOU FOR REAL?

I KEEP ASKING MYSELF: ARE YOU FOR REAL?
I OPEN MY MOUTH TO SPEAK, BREAKING THE SEAL,

Gary Michael Ruddick

FEELING FOR YOU IN RETURN, SPIRITUALLY
TRYING TO GET A FEEL,
THINGS ARE DIFFERENT TO US; NOW THAT'S
PART OF THE DEAL,
SOME THINGS ARE NOT THE SAME AS TO
YOU, THEY ARE UNREAL,
EVEN EATING FROM A PLATE SOME
CREATURES YOU SHOULD NOT KILL,
YET, EVEN PEOPLE ARE SLAUGHTERED AND
IT'S DONE JUST FOR A THRILL,
AND YET, YOU CANNOT GIVE THE DEAD A
REPRODUCTIVE PILL,
THE DEAD DO NOT RECEIVE A WELCOMING
BELL,
FOR MANY OF THEM ARE NEVER TO RETURN
FOR THAT IS THE PATH OF HELL,
WHAT BECOMES OF THEM IS SOMETHING I
CAN NEVER TELL, FOR THAT IS NOT A PLACE
THAT I BELONG TO OR DO I DWELL,
OR PATHS HAVE ONLY JUST BEGUN AND I
DO NOT BID YOU FAREWELL,
FOR ONE DAY I KNOW YOU WILL HELP ME TO
MAKE ME SAFE AND WELL,
FOR CHILDISHLY YOU ARE A BIT OF A TINKER
BELL,
AND I SHALL ALWAYS WISH YOU WELL,
FOR YOU WERE THE QUEEN ON THE LUCKY
PENNY THAT I FLIPPED INTO THE WISHING
WELL,
SOMETIMES LIFE IS A LIVING HELL,

GARY RUDDICK POEMS

I MOVE FROM RUNE TO ROOM AS IF IT WERE A LIVING CELL,
THERE HAVE BEEN TIMES WHEN I HAVE TRIPPED AND FELL,
BUT YOU HAVE UP RIGHTED ME WITH THE WIND IN MY SAIL, I HAVE, FOR THE MAJORITY OF MY ADULT LIFE, BEEN LOCKED UP IN A JAIL,
UNBEKNOWN TO ME, ONE DAY, A STORY I WOULD TALE,
I DO APOLOGISE FOR BECOMING PSYCHOTICALLY FRAIL,
BUT MY FRIEND SOME WALLS I JUST COULD NOT SCALE,
NEITHER DO I EAT FROM A GRASS'S BAIL,
I DO NOT EAT FOOD THAT IS OLD AND STALE,
SOMETIMES I FEEL OLD AND PALE,
I CAN NO LONGER ASK A JUDGE TO GRANT ME BAIL,
YET I'LL TRY NOT TO SHOUT AND WAIL,
IM NOT A DRINKER REALLY, SO I DON'T NEED THE ALE,
BUT I'M BLINDED LIKE SAMSON SO I NEED MY TAIL,
I SHALL RETURN IN STATURE AS LARGE AS A WHALE,
MY FILE I HOPE WITH YOU SHALL GROW, MY FRIEND IT SHOULD NOT BE FOR SALE,
FOR ONLY WITH YOU SOME THINGS I MAY TELL,

FOR THE WORLD IS MADE UP WITH A SINGLE
SPELL,
THAT IS THE TRUTH OF THE HOLY GRAIL,
DO NOT THINK THAT I AM ON THE GHOSTS'
TRAIN ABOUT TO BE DERAILED,
FOR IN MY MIND AND ON MY HAND MY LIFE IS
IN DETAIL,
AS WE ALL COME FROM THE SAME MAJESTIC
LIVING CELL,
SO FOR NOW I'LL BID YOU GOOD LUCK AND
FAREWELL.

GARY RUDDICK POEMS

CASTING MY SHADOW

Strange how the sunshine always casts a shadow,
Yet cupid flies through the air on the wings of a
sparrow,

Flowing from his heart the emotions of his arrow,
Strange how his heart line is so very narrow,

He will always bring you joy for tomorrow,
Please wipe away your tears of sorrow,

Love is something from another that you could
never borrow,
For the heart and soul search for something that
isn't hollow,

My path, my darling, no one can follow,
For if you could you would know about tomorrow,

My shadow is in the form of many colours,
For each shade have sisters and brothers,

In my life I have loved many others,
For in my path there are distant lovers,

Platonically, I love him as my brother,
Respectfully, I love you as my mother,

If I had the power I would ask you to become my
lover,

Gary Michael Ruddick

For in my heart I can no longer choose another,

The colour that I cast in my die is of the brightest purple light,
For there is no shadow that's more powerful than it in the night,

For that is the colour of the shepherd's delight,
For it is at this time that the gods and goddesses unite,

Far too long, man has struggled and had to fight,
It seems to me that no one has the answer to put it right,
Strange how many do not see the light,
For there are too many wrongs and not enough rights,

Not enough candles and not enough lights,
I wonder, at times, how the stars always hold their own light,

Never in the daylight have you seen the starlight,
For they move around the system into the silent night,

Never casting a shadow over the sunlight,
Always shimmering in the moonlight,

Do you recall when you first saw your first colour of light?

GARY RUDDICK POEMS

Was it in the form of the rainbow up there in the twilight?

Was it the gleam when your baby saw you for the first time with its eyesight?
For to that child you will always be that piece of light,

When you put them to sleep and hug them ever so tight,
Kissing them innocently, and saying to them gently: "god bless and goodnight".

Maybe one day with love and guidance our children will put the world to rights,
Open the heavens and show those that are lost to open their eyes to the paths into the light,

Time can only tell if our lives were the fight,
My friend, for now I will leave on my light,

The hands of time are joined on the left and the right,
If you put them together and pray there is no need to fight,

Who knows, maybe one day in the future things just may turn out alright.

Gary Michael Ruddick

GARY RUDDICK POEMS

CHRISTMAS

When you were young you were my own bundle of
joy
It didn't matter if you were a girl or a boy
For you were worth more than my favourite toy
When I feel love with your mother there was never
any ploy
To you, my child, I would offer the universe,
For you, on your birthday I shall remove a curse,
For a life wasn't meant for a black hearse,
The rainbow is for a gold purse,
For you have sang & read every verse,
My son you are a child of many
Yet you are my first,
For it was love, my child, that was your thirst,
That you gave your life to the earth,
My child, understand your every worth,
It is to you my child that I offer the earth,
It was you who gave your life to save the rest of
us,
So Happy Birthday&, a very Happy Christmas,
This is a script from all of us,
Thank-you
So we offer you more than water and a crust,
For you shall never return to ashes or dust,
For you're still in love with us,
My son, Happy Christmas.

COME WHAT MAY

IN THE NIGHTS SKY AMONGST THE STARS A
PATH FOR YOU I SHALL PAVE,
IN THE WARMTH OF THE SUMMERS HEAT
FLOWERS I SHALL NURTURE AND WITH LOVE
RAISE,
YOUR KINDNESS AND COMMITMENT FOR
TRUTH AND UNDERSTANDING I SHALL
PRAISE,
MY EMOTIONS TOWARDS YOU, TIME COULD
NEVER HOPE TO ERASE,
THE BEAUTY AND KINDNESS THAT
OUTWARDLY AND INNOCENTLY SHOW,
THE HONESTY AND MATURITY THAT IS
WITHIN YOU SHALL GROW AND GROW,
I SHALL LOVE YOU FOREVER I HOPE AND
PRAY THAT, THAT IS SOMETHING THAT YOU
MUST ALREADY KNOW,
I DREAM THAT YOU SHALL NEVER LET THAT
THOUGHT GO,
THEY DO SAY IN ANCIENT TIMES GONE BYE
THAT YOU REAP WHAT YOU SOW,
MY LOVE FOR A WOMAN NO LONGER HAS A
PLACE TO GO,
I KNOW THAT DEEP DOWN IN MY HEART
YOUR MIND WILL ALWAYS TELL ME NO,
MY FEELINGS OF LOVE FOR YOU I COULD
NEVER HAVE HIDDEN AND I HAD TO LET
THEM SHOW,

GARY RUDDICK POEMS

IN MY HEART FOR YOU THERE SHALL
ALWAYS BE A WARMTH A REASSURING
GLOW,
IN THE WINTER THE WARMTH THAT I FEEL
WOULD MELT THE COLDEST SNOW,
I WOULD FOREVER LOVE YOU CHERISH YOU,
HONOUR AND OBEY,
IF ONLY YOU WOULD LET ME THINGS WOULD
TURN OUT OKAY,
I SHALL LOVE YOU YESTERDAY TOMORROW
YET ILL LOVE YOU MORE TODAY,
THE LOVE I HAVE INSIDE OF ME FOR YOU
NOT EVEN A LIFE TIME OF THE EARTH
COULD MAKE IT FADE AWAY,
NO MATTER WHAT PEOPLE BEHIND CLOSED
DOORS WISH TO SAY,
I HAVE ALWAYS SAID COME WHAT MAY,
AS THE DARKNESS ENFOLDS THE DAY,
FOR YOU EACH NIGHT I ALWAYS REMEMBER
TO PRAY,
THAT YOU MAKE IT BACK TO THE LIGHT AT
THE BEGINNING OF EACH DAY,
IN MY DREAMS IS WHERE I HOPE THAT YOU
SHALL ALWAYS STAY,
I COULD NEVER FORGET YOUR KINDNESS I
HOPE THAT ONE DAY IT CAN BE REPAID,
FOR I AM NO LONGER LONELY OR AFRAID,
FOR SO LONG ON THE WRONG PATH I HAVE
STRAYED,
I REALISE THERE ARE TIMES WHEN IM SURE
THAT YOU ARE DISMAYED,

YET LIFE IS SOMETHING THAT CAN NEVER
BE REPLAYED,
EMOTIONS THOUGHTS CAN ALWAYS BE
RELAYED,
I TRUST AND LOVE YOU AND I KNOW THAT
WITH YOU I COULD NEVER BE BETRAYED,
WITH THE KNOWLEDGE THAT YOU HAVE
TAUGHT ME ONE DAY I MAY BE SAVED,
FOR WITHOUT YOU I SURELY WOULD HAVE
LONG AGO BEEN IN SLAVED,
LONG AGO THE PRESENCE OF MYSELF
WOULD HAVE BEEN CRUELLY ERASED,
YET A PATH FOR ME I DREAM THAT YOU MAY
ONE DAY PAVE,
IN ANOTHER LIFETIME WAY BEYOND THE
GRAVE.

GARY RUDDICK POEMS

DAY DREAMING

If I were to be born, once again could you wash me with oils under a cool mountain spring?
Could you with your soft and soothing musical voice gently for me sing?
Dreamily to the sweetness and protectiveness I am lulled to sleep trustingly to you do I cling?
Knowingly that the warmth of your heart shall always bring,
With you as my mother I feel that could never hope to ask for anything,
For the moments that we have lovingly and sacredly shared together with me, you are all and everything,
For as a child right from the beginning from my heart you pulled much more than a few stings,
For on my head of hair you did place a crown proclaiming someday in a dream that I would become a king,
Faraway in the distance the sound of wedding bells did ring,
In time, you said be quiet mature patient and wise and I could learn through time how to love many sacred things,
YOU stated that if I was kind and gentle maybe the birds to me would sing,
Until such a time you would guide and shelter me under your wings,
Only on that I promise that this time on earth I would not take a thing,

With that oath, I swore to you that only love and honour to you would I bring,

On my hand you placed upon my finger a band of precious yellow metal, which you said was a trust ring,

If I remained, as true to you as you promised you would be to me good fortune it would one day bring,

You spoke with truth trust and an immense knowledge of wisdom and to those words I did cling,

You spoke with strength experience and what I had heard from you today I must take heed and never tell a living thing,

The trust you were bestowing upon me was fit for a high king,

With that bond of love and trust between his mother and her kin,

Emotions deep inside brought tears of joy from within,

Dreaming of the time wishfully pondering if those dreams will one day begin,

Now as the daylight begins to pass and the night lets it self once again back in,

Reality once more again begins to return and I have to take it all in,

Yet that is the price you have to pay if you choose to commit a sin,

You can walk on water but be careful that the ice isn't to thin,

GARY RUDDICK POEMS

For even if you can swim the shock will freeze you
right through your skin,
If your sin is too heavy you will breathe the ice-
cold water in,
Down in the dark and murky waters of Hades the
coldness will get through to you from within,
A time shall come when it will be your nightmare
that shall begin,
Warning signs appear in your mind the night's chill
gets into you as you breathe the chill wind in,
Wondering what tomorrow dreams it might bring,
The passing thought that is floating before my
eyes is that this moment of reflection did not cost
a thing,
So wouldn't it be wise instead of taking isn't it time
whoever we may be started giving,
For we are not always going to be that of the
living,
Just think very briefly where are all those gone
before are they all accounted fore or is everybody
missing,
I wonder if there are other elements seeing, and
what about those that are silently hearing,
Who according to them is doing in their minds all
the speaking?
Who in the past has done what and is it their time
to fear,
For is your conscience once again from yesterday
reappearing,
Is your date with destiny suddenly unbearable?

Now is your fuddled mind through lack of drugs clearing?
Are you now focused and have you regained your bearings,
It does not matter if its jeans or a suit you are wearing,
It is just another tiresome tribunal hearing,
At the end of the day who's really caring,
For your taking the blame as you were to daring,
You should have kept quite instead of all that swearing,
At the end of the day, you were a lost lamb and you ended up bleating,
In a place like this it's a bit self-defeating,
All they entice you to do is come alone to the community meeting,
All they do there is constant bickering and swearing,
You get the odd one in the corner laughing and snickering,
Then there's his sidekick who does all the mimicking,
No matter where you go in life it will always be inflicting,
Therefore, life can be a wicked thing,
It all depends on what you are dealing,
Word of advice just very careful what you are stealing,
There are some brutal beatings,
For there are those that have no feelings,

GARY RUDDICK POEMS

However, how do you put a stop to the meaningless killings?
For a woman or a Childs life can never return through spiritual healing,
I may even know more than you think with my introvert thinking,
Every word rearranged has a different meaning,
However, I am not writing to sound demeaning,
All I'm doing is a bit of explaining,
For doing so I'm getting an education is what I'm gaining,
So if I'm not sleepiness it's because I'm refraining,
F or at times this place does your mind in,
In addition, the pills are one not all that rewarding,
Therefore, I hope on some of you it's dawning,
If you choose to abuse yourself, you may end up dead, as you do not from death get a second calling,
So if you think that is a kind of warning,
Just wait until the flames start your body warming,
FORGIVE ME I don't intend to be charming,
HOWEVER, it is still early in the morning,
Therefore, if I carry on it might sound boring,
In addition, I do not intend to end up yawning,
As before you know it ill next be snoring,
So good day and good morning.

DEEP IN THOUGHT

Sitting here in the dark with only confusion in my mind,
Asking myself, why did life have to be so unkind?
Silencing my deep inner fears, knowing that I no longer have to look behind,
Unknown people tracing my past-life hoping they might find something sinister.

Years have gone by and still they have nothing to report,
Strange how it's only for the stupid things that you get caught,
Looking at the blank faces, they weren't that well taught,
As for myself, I'm always deep in thought.

Looking over moments that I have sat with you wondering if you really were a godsend,
Wishing that just maybe you could perhaps one day become a true friend,
Yet in your line of work it would only be, let's just pretend,
I guess that a broken heart is something that you can't mend.

Wondering out loud should I continue shifting through emotions in my head, induced by drink and drugs my emotions are well and truly fed,

GARY RUDDICK POEMS

Clouds block out the vision of you, I'm no longer
listening to what you've said,
Condemned for something that you've read,

Invisible restraints restricting my dreams and
desires,
Chemically induced emotions, visions of you
dancing in the distant fire,
The soft gentle voice in the back of my mind telling
me that I still love you and it will always be you
that I desperately desire,
My mind doesn't accept the thought and now I'm
calling myself a liar.

Painstakingly searching through a passage in
time, trying to reclaim my long lost youth,
The drink and drugs, relationships were not really
that kind – looking in the mirror here's the image
of proof,
Smiling to myself I see the gap where as a child
there used to be a tooth,
My mind's silent once again; thoughts have stilled
themselves I wonder for now... if the unseen
voices have finally called a truce.

Thoughts of you calm me each night and every
day,
Now my mind no longer has the urge to go astray,
I get confused and reckless when you have to go
away,

Maybe that's the real reason why here is where, for the moment, I will stay.

GARY RUDDICK POEMS

FALLING INTO A DEEP SLEEP

I want to so somewhere that you can not speak,
I want to fall into an eternal sleep,
I want to lie down in the sea so deep,
I want to go where the trees don't creak,
I hope for me you will never seek,
Please promise me that you will not weep,
My mind has gone to deep,
Now is the right time for me to sleep,
For I see the shadows that try to creep,
Life these days has become too cheap,
Religion is worthless even a Christian to a sheik,
Everything is worth nothing so to speak,
If you understand this please do not speak,
For you are not the one that has been disposed of
by the beak,
The strength that I once was given disappears
each week,
I look in the mirror and I think I'm a freak,
Once I was strong now I am weak,
The future I see is only too bleak,
I will not be classed as one of the meek,
My skin is the colour of teak,
My body has grown old and now I creak,
Never has my life felt so cheap,
Nothing on this earth do I wish to reap?
No one and nothing do I seek,
I no longer understand the words you speak,
If you find me in a heap,
Do not try to wake me for I have gone to deep,

Gary Michael Ruddick

Please don't think of me as a lost sheep,
These are my last words on a sheet,
I have family, who once lived in Crete,
Maybe in another time and place I may let you meet,
My resting place is not that deep,
I shall hear you if you weep,
There are answers about a life that you should never sleep,
Please let me rest peacefully in my eternal sleep.

Love always
Your friend forever

GARY RUDDICK POEMS

FLIRTING IN BETWEEN INSANITY AND SANITY

Do you really understand the meaning of the term confidentiality?
If I were to whisper that I was in love with you desperately
Since the beginning of life I have desired you secretly
Now do you begin to understand the meaning of the term insanity?
So my love I am trying very hard to keep hold of my
Sanity,
For that my love is where I am today that is the state of my sanity,
Every time I set my eyes upon you I go all fidgety,
My emotions inside become all panicky.
The feelings that my body soul and mind present themselves inside of me come from the heart and I mean this honestly,
For the majority of my life I have lied and deceived most people dishonestly,
When I am in your presence I have listened and you have taught me about psychologically,
I feel at this moment that I have not wasted your time professionally,
Or have I invaded your personal space if so I apologise profusely,
As time revolves continually I hold you in the highest esteem and I swear to you truthfully

My feelings my feelings that I have now acquired for you are that of nothing more than that of a gentleman to that of a lady respectfully,

I shall not lie for there are moments that I have and always hope too to desire you and love you secretly,

Hopefully in another lifetime if you would consider the possibility that I could love you physically,

I would love you for as long as a man could earnestly not judge mentally and in all religiously,

My thoughts are honest and pure for I love you so very much spiritually,

I do not deny that my emotions have wandered where we entwined physically,

Forgive me my friend if I have breached the limitations of your boundaries,

In my dreams one the names that you go by is that of the innocence of purity,

When I dive into the crystal blue waters of your eyes the thoughts of you are heavenly,

My thoughts of you have and shall not ever reach the depths of depravity,

Neither have they been in any such way has my mind come across as derogatively,

I do see our minds working against one another one challengingly,

For that would surely change our outlook on and I would not want to for us to look at one another awkwardly,

GARY RUDDICK POEMS

I have and always shall look up to you in admiration,
I also think I'm assured that we have respected one another accordingly,
At this moment in our time I will try to keep a hold onto my sanity,
For sometimes it is so very hard to return to normality,
 Maybe I am to blame for my own stupidity,
My dear friend I finish this where I started and that is where I started thankfully,
That is I have not touch with my sanity or my reality,
Yours lovingly and faithfully religiously and trustingly.

Love,

Gary
xxxxx

****

For I do not have the guidance nor the ability to train my mind naturally in the art s of relaxation,
The words I put down on paper have entered my mind in their own formation,
So for when you are reading this I am holding my breathe with a somewhat nervous anticipation,
I can now look back over my life at times now with more than enough painful and also happy emotions,

And now I look into the clear waters and because of the calmness and tranquillity of my mind I do not need to question anymore my own reflection,

There have been at times in my life when I have had only myself in the form of some sort of conversation,

There are moments when I have had to use my own intuition,

And there are issues far too many for me to even mention,

As a child I always dreamed that I would when I grew up I would rid the world of all its man made pollution,

For I'm sure that there are many countries with money and power that if only they were to use it on trying to achieve a round the globe a more peaceful solution,

For many years we as a race of people have imbedded from our ancestors in us belong to one of the oldest religions,

There are those that due to nature's unique process of our departure or our elimination, naturally or by some foreign terrorists' organization,

And there are those that that have given love time money and even their lives to maintain our children have a chance to build on our very foundations,

That one day some where I hope in the not to distant future we could one day through listening to each other we could once again have a peaceful and united civilization,

So if there are those that are in a position and intelligent enough and have the dedication,

To bring peace to every religion and to every independent nation,

For the life of an innocent child's love and presence here on earth you could never regain their innocence beauty by offering those unfortunate to have lost a loved one, compensation,

And if those that now have to spend their lives in total isolation,

There are those who survive in the underground or as they call it: the segregation,

Because we can not be bothered with all the aggravation,

So to tell you the truth I have only come here to this institution,

Maybe just may be I'm looking for some sort of salvation,

So do you not think that I've long passes the date to be referred to as the new admission?

Who knows after reading this you just might become a born again Christian,

Just please don't ask me to tell you about all the different editions,

For now though this closes a chapter in my life and hopefully I can one day return to normality and to do what I have always dreamed of doing and that's to venture on a space mission,

But knowing me ill end up on some crazy expedition,
Sat somewhere in the freezing cold fishing and wishing.

GARY RUDDICK POEMS

GARY'S
RESIDENTS.
PLEASE
KNOCK
GENTLY
BEFORE
LOOKING
AND
ENTERING.
MUCH
OBLIGED.
NO.7

DEAR MOTHER

If showered you with the stars from above,
Would you always promise to show me true love?
If I returned to you as a fox cub,
Would I once again have to wear the glove?
To me you were always my white dove,
And to me there is no purer symbol of love,
If I showered you with all my love,
Would you believe me if I told you the laws from
above,
If I reigned down upon you all of my charm,
Would the world one day disarm?
I may be a lamb yet I was not raised on a farm,
Do I once again enter a crypt only to be
embalmed?
You honestly and truthfully know that I could never
harm you physically,

For I love you mother innocently, desperately and spiritually,
As your son you loved and adored me magically and tenderly,
Little did you know from you I inherited a little bit of your wizardry?
It was never my intension to wander off my path and go astray,
Yet I did not wish to return to the oats and hay,
I shall never lose my way for you know I have never been afraid,
Mother my soul could never be enslaved,
My light shall never diminish nor shall it be mislaid,
On my heart your name has been engraved,
My soul therefore is no longer enraged,
Mother for the kind and loving friend that you have always been I realize that my soul never needed to be saved,
My love for you cannot and never shall be ever erased,
For my silent thoughts on this day shall tonight from me be prayed?
There are mother thoughts and feelings that need not be written on a page,
And today is a very special day, for you have reached a lovely age,
But I do not need to remind you my precious mother,
I hope and pray that you shall be here in my heart forever...

GARY RUDDICK POEMS

HAPPY BIRTHDAY MOTHER.

LOVE YOUR LOVING SON

GARY
XXXXX

MANY A PERSON HAS LEFT US IN A PUFF OF SMOKE!

It all began with that first intake of the unknown mysterious white and grey innocent smoke.
You breathe in deeply as it's your first time, unbeknown to you it shall not be your last, therefore you begin to cough and choke.
Once you begin it shall take a grip so hard on you that you will lose everything and you could end up broke,
When you're no longer satisfied with your usual daily intake, you will move onto the next best thing, surely it's the right thing to do of course its dope!
You enjoy the sensation, alas the paranoia. Silently you are unaware of your down fall, you continue to smoke. So I shall bid you my friend, farewell, for I witnessed many individuals swing from a rope,
Once you have escalated to that level of despair in your mind there is no longer any hope,
If your mind is still stable and in tune with reality you will most probably continue to take!
With the cost of living and your addiction can you still keep your head afloat?
You now have a desire through your craving to move up a level and sniff that lovely fine white powder. For in your mind this is the 'real thing' coke!

GARY RUDDICK POEMS

I do not intend to speak a single word. For it was in your mind that the voice spoke,

Your mind has some how been destroyed, the power of the crystal amphetamines and your deepest fears have awoke,

Will the voice that now permanently remains in your mind soothe you, or will it torment you? For now you pray silently and desperately, for you imagine that it is the pope.

You do not realize that the reality that you once knew is no more. You are no longer able to cope!

Your whole body, even your existence has sadly been broke.

Thinking back over the years if I remember rightly, you were a great bloke,

Now your head and your heart are rushing with adrenaline, please slow down for you may have a stroke!

Your addiction takes over; the urge is too strong,

You are going to do the ultimate, your going to have a poke!

I suppose that once you reach this stage life no longer seems appealing and at the end of the day you cannot afford to take life as a joke!

In the beginning the sensation of every individual drug may feel good, No matter how high you float,

You must be aware that it could be the illegal substances that you are thinking of testing and the tears that will be cried shall be of many.

The lump in the throat of those who loved you, the tears will fall openly and silently. For it is the living that are choked.

Isn't it strange how there are so many ways to build a fire!

I'm sure that when it comes to be our turn that the fire shall be well stoked.

At the end of the day, the choice is in your hands, you can say yes to drugs or you can say no!

It doesn't matter!

For we all go up in a blaze of flames of white and grey smoke!

All I can say is that the answer I am looking for is to say NO, I pray and I hope!

GARY RUDDICK POEMS

HEALING!

IN THE DARK FOR THE FIRST TIME IN MY
LIFE,
I AM ON MY KNEES HANDS TOGETHER AND
KNEELING,
DEEP DOWN INSIDE OF MYSELF I HAVE THIS
UNKNOWN FEELING,
THOUGHTS OF WHAT IF YOU OR I CAN
REMOVE THIS WITH NATURAL HEALING,

AS THE DAYS TURN INTO MONTHS YEARS
EVEN I HAVE THIS DEEP IMBEDDED FEELING,
THAT ONE DAY IN THE NOT TO DISTANT
FUTURE I MAY DECIDE THAT IT IS TIME THAT
I AM PREPARED TO START LEAVING,
I JUST PRAY THAT AS MY FRIEND YOU WONT
START GRIEVING,
THE LIGHT IN MY SOUL HAS ALREADY
STARTED RECEDING,

FOR MY MIND CAN NO LONGER ACCEPT THIS
ABNORMAL FEELING,
MY MIND IS TELLING MYSELF WAS THIS A
MERCY KILLING,
THERE ARE TIMES WHEN MY HEAD JUST
WON'T SPOT SPINNING,
PSYCHOLOGICALLY I AM NO LONGER
LOSING OR WINNING,

DO I FIGHT THE TEMPTATION TO MAKE A
NOOSE OUT OF A PIECE OF LINING,
THIS IS JUST TO SHOW THAT MY
ENDURANCE HERE ON EARTH IS THINNING,
IF YOU WERE HERE I WOULD WANT TO HOLD
YOU AS I THINK THE DARKNESS IS FINALLY
WINNING,
MAYBE I CAN RETURN AS A CHILD ONCE
MORE TO WHEN THE PLANETS WERE
SPINNING,

WHEN THE SEAS WERE CALM AND THE
MERMAIDS WERE SOFTLY SINGING,
FROM WAVE TO WAVE, YOU GODDESSES OF
THE SEA S TAUGHT ME THE ART OF
SWIMMING,
WHEN I DIVED FOR A PEARL YOU ALL WERE
SMILING
EVEN WHEN I RETURNED EMPTY HANDED
YOU JUST SAID KEEP ON TRYING,

FOR AT THE BOTTOM OF THE OCEAN THERE
IS A SILVER LINING,
FOR IT IS THE PATH OF THE MOON THAT YOU
SEE SHINING,
NEVER TO BRIGHT AND NEVER TO BLINDING,
SILENTLY TO THE STARS IT IS SECRETLY
REMINDING,
THAT ALL THE PLANETS ARE SLOWLY
UNWINDING,

GARY RUDDICK POEMS

IF YOU WERE TO GET TO CLOSE TO THE
LIGHTS IN THE CONSTELLATION THE
HORIZON THAT YOU WOULD SEE WOULD BE
AMASS OF LIGHTING,
FOR THE STARS ARE A PATH TO A
DIFFERENT OPENING,
YET HOW MANY RACES HAVE THOUGHT
ABOUT ELOPING,
I SIT HERE ON EARTH WAITING FOR YOU AND
SILENTLY AND SECRETLY HOPING,

THROUGH TIME AND SPACE, I WOULD GUIDE
YOU FROM PLANET TO PLANET HOPING
THAT TOGETHER, WE COULD SAVE THE
RACES,
EVEN THE UNBORN THOSE WHO STILL HAD
TO LEARN ABOUT THEIR AIRS AND GRACES,
WATCH THE SHINE IN THEIR EYES AND THE
SMILES PERMANENTLY ON THEIR FACES,
AS WE TOLD THEM ALL THE MAGICAL
PLACES AND ABOUT THE SACRED HOLY
PLACES,

WE COULD TAKE THEM THROUGH AT
DIFFERENT STAGES,
YOU COULD READ AND I WOULD TURN THE
PAGES,
TO TELL THEM THE HISTORY OF OUR WORLD
WOULD TAKE AGES,
FOR AT FIRST WE WOULD HAVE TO SHOW
THEM THE PICTURE PAGES,

FIRST WE WOULD HAVE TO EXPLAIN ABOUT
THE BALL OF FIRE IN THE SKY,
AND IF ONE DAY YOU GOT TO CLOSE IT
WOULD HURT YOU EYES,
AND YOU WOULDN'T WANT TO WEAR DARK
GLASSES AS THERE ARE THOSE WHO WILL
SAY ARE YOU IN DISGUISE,
HOWEVER, MAYBE YOU ARE HIDING YOUR
INTELLIGENCE? BUT IS THAT REALLY WISE,

SO REMOVE THEM FOR YOU MAY GET A
PLEASANT SURPRISE,
FOR OUT OF THE EARTH A ROSE MAY ARISE.

GARY RUDDICK POEMS

HERE I GO AGAIN

HAS IT EVER OCCURRED TO YOU THE
THOUGHTS THAT GO THROUGH YOUR BRAIN,
HAVE YOU EVER WONDERED IF IT'S EVERY
BODY ELSE THAT ARE INSANE,
MY THOUGHTS THEY SHALL NEVER
CONTAIN,
SPIRITUALLY I SHALL NEVER BE LOCKED UP
AGAIN,
FOR PHYSICALLY ALL YOU CAN DO IS
CONTAIN,
SURELY THEY MUST FEEL A SENSE OF
SHAME
AND I SHALL FETCH THAT CUP NEVER FEEL
THE SAME,
YOU PILLS WILL NEVER BRING THE CLOCK
BACK AGAIN,
FOR WHAT THEY DID WAS INSANE,
BUT THAT'S THE THOUGHT PROCESS OF
THEIR BRAIN,
TO WASH AWAY A LIFE DOWN THE DRAIN,
I ASK MYSELF TO THIS EARTH WHY HAVE I
CAME,
THE TRUTH IS IT WAS TO LOVE YOU ONCE
AGAIN,
THE EMOTIONS THAT RUN THROUGH MY
BRAIN,
MY LOVE YOU DO NOT UNDERSTAND MY
PAIN,

HERE I AM ALONE ONCE AGAIN,
I AM NOT ONE TO FEEL THE EMOTION OF
SHAME,
SO FROM THAT THOUGHT I SHALL ABSTAIN,
THOUGHTS OF YOU RUNNING THROUGH MY
BRAIN,
MY FANTASIES OF YOU ARE NOW TRAINED,
I HOPE I DON'T COME ACROSS AS BEING
DERANGED,
IM NOT TO YOU I HOPE EVEN A LITTLE BIT
STRANGE,
HAS MY LOVE FOR YOU NOT YET REACHED
YOUR RANGE,
YOU SAID YOU WERE STRICT MADAME
AMANDA,
DOES THAT MEAN YOU USE A CANE?
I DON'T USUALLY DO SEXUAL PAIN,
BUT IF IT WAS YOUR WANT I WOULD PLAY
YOUR GAME,
AS LONG AS YOU DIDN'T WANT ME TO
DRESS AS A DAME,
FOR AT THE MOMENT I DON'T HAVE A MAINE,
IS THIS BEGINNING TO SOUND INSANE,
BUT MY LOVE YOU ARE NO PLAIN JANE,
SO FOR ME FALLING IN LOVE WITH I AM NOT
TAKING THE BLAME,
I ONLY PRAY THAT ONE DAY OUR PATHS
BECOME THE SAME, FOR YOU I SHALL HOLD
MORE THAN A FLAME,
IN YOUR PROFESSION I KNOW IT GOES
AGAINST THE GRAIN,

GARY RUDDICK POEMS

YET COULD NT YOU SECRETLY LOVE ME THE
SAME,
FOR YOUR IMAGE IS DEEPLY IMBEDDED IN
MY BRAIN,
MY LOVE MY HEART CANNOT HOLD THIS
PAIN,
FOR TONIGHT I AM ALONE AGAIN,
SILENTLY I SHALL SLEEP NOW WHISPERING
YOUR NAME,
GOODNIGHT AND I LOVE YOU AND GOD
BLESS.

****

HERE IS WHERE I PLEAD
I ASK YOU MY FRIEND
WOULD YOU BE WITH ME UNTIL THE END,
WOULD TO ME YOUR LIGHT COULD YOU
LEND,

MY LOVE FOR YOU IS THAT OF A FRIEND,
THAT MY DEAR I DO NOT PRETEND,
MY LIFE LINE I THINK MAY ONE DAY END
THAT TO YOU I DO NOT PRETEND,

THE TEARS THAT I SILENTLY AND OPENLY
SHED,
ARE FOR THOSE CHILDREN THAT ARE LONG
FORGOTTEN,

YET IN HEAVEN THEIR NAMES EACH DAY
ARE JOYFULLY READ,
SOME HAVE SADLY PASSED AWAY BEFORE
THEY REACHED THE AGE TO SLEEP IN A
BED,

SOME BABIES RETURN TO THEIR MAKER NO
LARGER THAN A LITTLE TED,
I ASK MYSELF WHY COULDN'T YOU OF
TAKEN ME INSTEAD,
FOR DAY AFTER DAY I STRUGGLE FOR
SURVIVAL IN MY HEAD,
WHEN A BABY PASSES THOUGH THE LAND
OF THE LIVING MY HEART ONCE AGAIN
FEELS LIKE LEAD,

FOR WE ALL MUST ENTER THE SECRECY OF
THE DEAD,
I NO LONGER FEEL OR ENJOY THE
LONELINESS OF MY BED,
AND CLOSING MY EYES IS SOMETHING I
DREAD,
FOR MY LIFELINE IS HANGING ON BY THE
SILK OF A SPIDERS THREAD,

IF MY TEARS WERE TO APPEAR IN THE
COLOUR OF RED,
COVERING ME FROM FOOT TO MY HEAD,
WOULD YOU REMEMBER THE BOOKS THAT
YOU LONG AGO ONCE READ,

GARY RUDDICK POEMS

WOULD YOU GENTLY CLOSE MY EYES AND
DECLARE THAT I WAS DEAD,

I DO REALISE AT TIME S SOME OF THE
THINGS THAT TRANSPIRE OUT OF MY HEAD,
ARE NOT ALWAYS MEANT AS THEY WERE
SAID,
AND I HOPE AND PRAY YOU HAVE BY ME NOT
BEEN MISLEAD,
FOR YOU MY FRIEND THERE HAS NEVER
BEEN A BAD THOUGHT FOR YOU INSIDE MY
HEAD.

You're a bit of my history and you want to be a
part of me

We could be a he or a tree

A piece of just you and me and I hope you won't
look down on me

For I had you down for the top of the Christmas
tree

If only you know what you do to me

I'd give you a leaf from my evergreen tree

For with me baby we would be history

Don't tell me honey you could disagree

So why don't you come and climb on me?

But you've got to set me free

And I'll treat you like a Royal Bee

So Do You?

My love, open your eyes or can't you see?

Open up your eyes and come to me

For here I am on my knees

Come on beautiful, let's join trees

Let's get our hands together and I'll say please.

GARY RUDDICK POEMS

HOME

Inside of you, there is more than just skin and bone,
For inside your mind is where you are at home,
You have peace of mind when you are on your own,
Sometimes you can only find solace when you are alone,
My saying is that your temple is also your throne,
There are no boundaries you can go anywhere if you like to roam,
Careful though as if you wander too far to soon you could finish up under a headstone,
Believe me that I is something that I do condone,
For if that were to occur there would not be anyone left at home,
Then again are there some of yours that are not alone,
For the sound of your voice is not of your usual tone,
Then again, it may be the rattle of your bones,
But you know what happens when he who throws stones,
Yet its never just one for they're not man enough on their on own,
For past events have already been shown,
Many a die has been thrown,
It is usually at the little defenceless garden gnome,
However, magically he could stand up on his own,
For on his mead he wears his wizard's cone,

In his bag of tricks, he carries his sticks and his bones,
Whence is in his home he reads his rune stones,
Remember the story? Give a dog a bone,
The truth is this little dog always used to crush it with a stone,
He would sit there until the wind had blown,
Waggling his tail head up off again him would roam,
For in the wind he would catch the sound of the trombone,
The music sang you must never again return home,
Fore the four kings and queens have long ago flown,
So now my little gnome your temple is made of stone,
For not even the sound of the trees creak bend and moan,
Will you let a soul into your sacred home?
For only you control what you do on your own,
Therefore, if you are sat there my friend s and you hear a woman's voice moan and groan,
You know she is playing with my bone,
If she shrieks with a very high pitched tone,
You do realize some games you do not play alone,
There are some things that I do not condone,
If you are a man, do not blow another's trombone,
For that turns my heart to solid stone,
History and fate have for centuries already shown,

GARY RUDDICK POEMS

That a man and a woman forever together long ago learned,
That it is for each other that they yearn,
That is why a man has his sacred sperm,
Therefore, the love and trust of a woman he has to earn,
Those that are to young one day will understand and if you are lucky, you might get your turn,
Promise me though that you will not be burned,
For love wasn't meant to carry any form of germ,
Yet I cannot comprehend why there are those that will not learn,
In the early stages of earth's natural life, you were only a little fern,
You were of the family the evergreen so that in the heat of the sun you would not burn,
Now I wonder patiently in which direction the wheels of the zodiac table shall now turn,
In which age will you try to do a u-turn?
What religion will you next remember of old and relearn,
Alternatively, whose is the next to be removed and overturned?
What race next is going to be spurned?
Cannot the lives of those lost through war and famine maybe one day magically secretly to those that have lost them be, returned?
WHY do the laws of nature have to be so cruel and so stern?
If to our scriptures of the ancient ones we were to return,

Would one day your guidance and your light again in the heavens burn

What sacrifice would the elements of life require in return?

How if ever your love for us once again could we earn,

Would the body of a caution inflamed in the most powerful element of those that were chosen since the hands of time turned,

Were their ashes placed in a sacred and holy urn?

For man and woman were to holy in the beginning for the worm,

I wonder which race and religion shall ever find the truth or will they never beckon,

For if you choose one day to return to your heavenly home, Would you could you promise that you would never leave us as we are still children if the truth be known,

Deep down no one likes to be left on his or her own,

Has it come to that age once more where nature and time have once more shown?

That we as the human race will one day be overthrown,

BY an element on this earth that has never before been known,

If by chance of fate we have in the sacred Garden of Eden through wisdom ignorance or just a thirst for knowledge this earth we have outgrown,

GARY RUDDICK POEMS

Show us the way towards another of your moonstones,
For if, you really are that smiling little garden gnome,
Why do you not come to our humble home?
For the age has passed when the architects first laid the stones,
Those that are the foundations of Rome,
At some stage all of the white candles will have been blown,
If those lights in your constellation were not a true reflection of your love that we deeply yearn,
Then I think in my mind there is nothing more here on earth to learn,
I've said my peace in my mind now it is your turn.
The path that you once walked on your footprints is no longer traceable so therefore I now walk alone,
My element in my soul shall for you always burn,
Just in case perhaps one day you choose to return?
Until whenever my child for you I shall always yearn,
Where ever your spirit has long ago flown,
I pray the right way you are shown and that is your way home.
FOR MY DEAR FRIEND, Gillian MAY YOUR SONS ANA YOUR DAUGHTERS ALWAYS FIND THE LIGHT ON THEIR PATH THROUGH LIFE AND THAT THEY ENJOY EVERY MOMENT OF THEIR YOUNGER YEARS FOR LIFE WITH

YOUR CHILDREN SHALL LAST A LIFE TIME.
YOUR BOND CAN ONLY GROW AS TIME GOES
BY; FOR NATURE HAS A WAY OF BRINGING
LOVED ONES BACK TO THE MOTHERS NEST
X.
WHERE YOU'RE KING WILL WAIT WITH HIS
WINGS OPEN WITH HIS HEART BEATING IN
HIS CHEST,
FOR YOU MY CHILD WILL ALWAYS BE
HEAVENLY BLESSED.

GARY RUDDICK POEMS

I HAVE NO REGRETS

Over the years I have had more than enough time
to reflect,
So I shall put this on paper before I forget,
I don't understand why you have become so
politically correct,
Every fortnight a chemical in my butt you forcibly
inject,
To tell the truth I feel like a scientists pet,
The day it due I begin to fret,
As really I want to stick it in your damned neck,
It's only then that I begin to reflect,
But I would rather cuss you off its politically
correct,
I wonder who's going to do it next,
I see those induced and they are all now wrecked,
Greasy hair and hen pecked,
Another lost soul society rejects,
I don't have a mobile so it's my own personal text,
I just hope my spelling is all correct,
I have my own copy so I know where there kept,
The truth is I never know what I intend to write
next,
I suppose its something that you have to accept,
As under the carpet our inner thoughts are swept,
Another session with the nurse my mental state
correct,
Pen in hand more lies I expect,
Looking into my eyes you never are direct,

Listening to my emotions you kid yourself that my situation you can accept,
You don't really understand me for we haven't and never shall get to that depth,
My only wish is that it was somewhere else that we had meet,
Deep down I have only one regret,
That is with you I had of taken a bet,
That what ever you tell me I will never accept,
For there are doubts long imbedded that you don't accept,
Then again you're politically correct,
Myself I'm always the suspect,
Strange you don't even know me yet,
Something that only I and my shadow secretly have kept,
To me though you were never a fret,
For you soothed me when my eyes were wet,
This isn't the place to have any regrets,
For meeting you was something that I didn't expect,
So the truth is the years gone by I have no regrets.
As my life is far from over yet,
Yet thinking of you there could never be a next,
Wondering for a moment I guess my fate was hexed,
The truth is I should be vex,
Yet I have no regrets.

GARY RUDDICK POEMS

I WANT TO SHARE IN YOUR SEXUALITY

As a child I learned early about my masculinity,
One day I dreamed I would find a girl who in time
would show me her femininity,
Together we would learn about each other's
sexuality,
What we had dreamed of would be innocent just
out of curiosity,
Our desires now could become a possibility,
No longer alone our minds lost in confusion and
fantasy,
Remembering your touch, the feel of your tongue
entwined with mine my heart beating ecstatically,
Memories of you holding me close, stroking my
stomach and chest seductively,
Whispering and soothing me gently whispering to
me ever so softly,
Brushing my hair out of my eyes playfully,
Smiling and laughing at me, with me joyfully,
Holding each other's hands innocently,
Looking deep into one another's eyes longingly,
Hugging each other close ever so tightly,
Talking to one another gleefully,
Touching parts of one another sheepishly,
Exploring sacred parts of each other secretly,
Looking into one another's eyes lovingly,
Biting one another's lips and tongue
mischievously,
Nibbling and tasting one another playfully,

Becoming tense and heated looking and touching each others bodies physically,

Loving you deeper than any other mythological goddess,

Loving you more honestly than any otter god spiritually,

Worshiping you honourably with all of my intimacy in privacy,

Forever praising you for all of eternity,

Longing to open up both honestly and emotionally.

To give myself to you whole heartedly,

Top always treats you gently lovingly and gently and tenderly,

Always to think and talk to you respectfully,

Never to talk about you indirectly or disrespectfully,

I could never demean you or belittle you psychologically,

I would always respect your beliefs respectfully and religiously,

I dream that one day I could share in your past and present life and your future holistically,

I would with you by my side grow together physically and psychologically,

Forever be by your side protectively,

Maybe one day we could in time become as one and share in your fertility,

For I have dreamed that I have drank and tasted from your sweetness of your virginity,

Now and forever your name in secret I shall call you heavenly and purity,

GARY RUDDICK POEMS

In my mind your beauty shall out shine any woman through out history,
I shall love you forever spiritually physically endlessly innocently for the rest of eternity.

****
*

I wonder
If you will ever really understand,
The force of a person's hand,
Why is it that some paths have to be damned?
Life sometimes is not always planned,

Many a person have been hanged,
Too many paths have been changed,
Drink and drugs have made them deranged,
The human race in my minds eye has now become very strange,

Do you justify putting a person in a cage?
For once in a lifetime getting into a rage,
Life is more than a calculated stage,
Some stories are never to be put down on a page,

Wisdom does not always come with age,
The light will not always follow the sunrays,
Sometimes the darkness shimmers and stays,

Gary Michael Ruddick

But in my mind that's to keep the truth away,

I wonder if spiritually I've flown away,
Was I really that little moggy who turned into a stray?
I'll be gone tomorrow but I'm here with you today,
I really needed to see you if that's okay,

Sometimes I wonder if I'm getting old and my mind has frayed,
Have I travelled to deep got trapped and enslaved,
Will the books of yesterday ever be obeyed?
It seems that in life no one is afraid,

I suppose that's the way that we were made,
I don't suppose it really matters anymore about yawed,
I do wonder firstly if you're okay,
For the moment that's the way my mind will stay,

I you could only take some time out and search into yourself; you will learn so much about the real you than you knew before,
It would be wise for me to explain that on your journey through life you are more than likely going to stumble and fall,
For I know you are strong and proud so this friend is what I shall tell you hold your head high and walk tall,
If at some stage in your career for whatever the reason my friend all you need do is call,

GARY RUDDICK POEMS

There have been stages in our past we have been locked inside four square walls,

Personally from my eyes under cover of darkness I have let the tears fall,

I have seen and heard many a mans spirit crumble and break, too many men crawl,

All through and around the system I have read their names and other writing scratched upon the wall,

Unfortunately, there are some that are. May they rest in peace no longer with us, for they only have the courage to shout and bawl.

Most of us try and do it silently and peacefully behind the iron door,

There are times when some of us are left naked and bloodied cuffed upon the floor,

Sadly they're a few that for some reason were not strong enough inside and took their life inside the prison wall,

As time goes bye you get thinking that you've seen it all now, for now you know that it's all been done before,

They even try to get you to submit by asking you to lock your self in behind your door,

When your entombed alive in a room it gets to you right down to the core,

Some of us used to train physically psyching our selves up as if were going to war,

For who knows what will happen next time they open your door,

New faces come and go every body gets asked what your name is? Where you from? And what are you in for? And how long? Every body knows the score,

There are those that have never been in the system before,

Some look at you with fear and terror in their eyes you can always the ones that are dodgy so you keep your distance for they make you sick and your skin begins to crawl,

For they attack women and the innocent and small,

You watch them sliver away to their pit and curl into a protective ball,

Things like that have become protected species that are guarded; I wonder how people are fooled?

Now do you wonder some of us are psychologically at war?

Yet at the end of the day it would be us that were punished if we had a brawl,

So some how we have to turn of our natural thoughts and emotions and wait silently for the lights out call,

There have been times when I wished I could have borrowed Freddie's claw

 For I think its time now that I my name to the wall?

I do hope that you realize now? And not later that I am not a fool,

I just do not understand why some people get wrapped in cotton wool,

GARY RUDDICK POEMS

Ana the things they do in their minds they think it's cool,

And at the end of the day were all made to look like fools,

And they get all the comfort s that are made available to them in the NHS hospitals,

And that it's all to do with their past and its psychological,

Forgive me if I come across as hypocritical,

Most of them do what they do because there sick nasty and spiteful,

So therefore they are punished to such an extent that they should never get the chance to destroy the opposite sex the old the young and the beautiful,

According to laws well before our time it was mans law, that they were made to beg and crawl,

I only regret that I wished I had studied law,

For there are some of us that know the score,

Deep in my bosom there is pounding like never before,

If I were to raise my voice it would be that of a lions roar,

IF I am still here when the winter rains begin to fall,

When I one day return to society and the gloves once again shall cover my paw,

Alas if fate has decided that that I must spend an indefinite period behind the fall

From outside my door no longer must you call?

For around my self I will have once again an invisible wall.

NAFF RESPECT.
GARY   M   RUDDICK.

20 6 2004

PS. I wonder how long the mothers and fathers will let the law decide what the deterrent is that will stop some crimes? For not even death would stop those capable and they don't even feel shame, so please AMANDA leave me out of the debate as like you said its sad.

You will always be fighting a war with the mind, everyone is a player of some form or another, the question is... if given the proper guidance any child can become a champion for all it takes is patience and determination, and the right people around at the right time.

GARY RUDDICK POEMS

IF I WERE TO GIVE YOU A PIECE OF MY
HEART,
WOULD YOU PROMISE NOT TO TEAR IT
APART,
THERE WILL BE MOMENTS WHERE I DO NOT
KNOW WHERE TO START,
MY FEELINGS FOR YOU ARE ONLY JUST
SURFACING AND THEY COME FROM AN
ANGELS HARP,

THERE HAVE BEEN MOMENTS WHEN I HAVE
SO DESPARATELY NEEDED A FRIEND,
EVEN I HAVE TRIED TO BRING MY LIFE TO AN
END,
SO MY FEELINGS FOR YOU AND OF YOU
SHALL NEVER COME TO AN END,
FOR THESE I HOPE ARE COMFORTING
WORDS OF I HOPE OF A CLOSE FRIEND,

THERE HAVE BEEN TIMES IN THE SHORT
TIME THAT WE HAVE SPOKEN TO ONE
ANOTHER AND MADE EACH OTHER SMILE,
THERE HAVE BEEN THE LITTLE BIT OF
SADNESS THAT YOU HAVE CRIED FOR A
LITTLE WHILE,
YET YOU HAVE YOUR AIRS AND YOUR OWN
BEAUTIFUL STYLE,
SO FOR THIS MOMENT IN THE PASSAGE OF
OUR LIVES CAN I LOVE YOU FOR A LITTLE
WHILE,

MY HEART AND SOUL I SHALL FOR YOU PUT
DOWN ON MANY PAGES
FOR FRIENDSHIP AND LOVE HAS TO GO
THROUGH MANY STAGES,
LOVE FOR SOME WILL TAKE FOREVER FOR
US IT COULD BE IN THE EARLY STAGES,
LOVE IS VERY EMOTIONAL AND IT HAS TO
BEGIN AT A PERSONS
EARLY AGES,

THERE ARE MOMENTS WHEN WE ALL GO
THROUGH THE FEELINGS OF STRESS,
THINKING BACK TO YESTERDAY AT TIMES
WILL GET MANY PEOPLE A LITTLE BIT
DEPRESSED,
IF YOU MY FRIEND NEED TO GET YOUR
EMOTIONS OF YOUR CHEST,
I AM ONLY A MOMENT AWAY YOU CAN PUT
PEN TO PAPER FOR THAT SHOULD PUT
YOUR MIND AT REST,

EVERY MAN WOMAN AND CHILD HAS GODS
OWN CREST,
JUST REMEMBER NATASHA YOU ARE AND
ALWAYS SHALL GOD BLESSED,
YOU MUST PROMISE ME THAT YOU WONT
PUT YOUR SOUL TO THE TEST,
FOR IF YOU DECIDE TO I SHALL NEVER BE AT
REST.

GARY RUDDICK POEMS

I WOULD LOVE TO HOLD YOU AND HUG YOU
TO MY CHEST,
I THINK MY LOVELY FRIEND YOU KNOW THE
REST,
TO FEEL THE SOFTNESS AND YOUR HEART
BEAT INSIDE YOUR BREAST,
DREAMING OF YOU FOR NOW I'LL RETURN
ALONE TO MY NEST.

Gary Michael Ruddick

IF YOU EVER!

If I am to be forever to lay down in eternal rest,
Please in my hands lay a four-leafed clover need I
say the rest,
Place over my heart a cross inside of my now
silent heart that which is inside of my chest,
All children are at some stage in their lives no
matter how long or short are forever and a day
blessed,
Many souls have been tormented even their lives
have been put to the test,
MORE than most will suffer others more than a
few their inner strength put to the limit even their
souls put to the test,
Many have been through the hardest walk of life
their spirits forever living in turmoil and insanity
and unrest,
Every child who walked swam or flew in the land
of this earth have always been welcome as a
guest,
There are those that are here at gods will and at
his request,
There are those that have given their lives through
believing in what is right for in their minds life is
much more than just a physical test,
If you continue to strive forward and always be
good you will not always be the best,
Long ago I fought for what I thought for what I
believed what was right, respectfully I held my
hands together to my chest,

GARY RUDDICK POEMS

Don't dwell on riches that might not even be
hidden in that secret chest,
Think about your history and your families crest,
Even if your families history is confusing and you
begin to feel a little bit stressed,
At some stage in your lifetime you may feel a bit
depressed,
I don't know your story but I'm not intending to put
you through the process,
Of going through the stages of the term that is
used called regress,
We all have a story about one thing or another
there are so many options it's easy to make a
guess,
So I shan't ask you any questions I wouldn't put
your mind through any paranoid test,
For the mind should after all these years be able
to put itself to rest,
There are times for that I have shed a tear for you
and there are moments we have spoken in jest,
Yet at the end of the day you are my father so its
time I put your mind at rest,
I hope that the years that you have here on earth
are blessed,
So happy birth day dad and I hope each drink you
put away in your mind you say! Gary god bless.
    Love, your son.

****

If you were a child again yet this time round you were rejected,

How do you suppose that child would be affected?

What if his emotions were misdirected?

And if the damage that was done could never be corrected,

What if the only way was for him to be forcibly and chemically injected?

Look around you for surely it is the foundations that you have built your society on that once again need to be inspected,

For I'm sure that it is not the child's behaviour or even his personality that to some show concern for haven't his thoughts and actions already been collected,

And all the traumas and events for most of his life all been put together and a picture and a pattern and all the pieces have been put together and they all connected,

What will be the next new drug to hide the scars bury the past block out the pain still the emotions and control the anger, of those void of any emotion sometimes guilt has been misdirected,

There are those whose minds that have been so badly infected,

And for the actions they have committed it is themselves that have weakened and been afflicted,

And in my eyes if it is the life of a women or a child from society you could only be evicted,

GARY RUDDICK POEMS

And even your breath sight and sound and hearing should be seriously,
Restricted,
And to take the life of any child is undeniably cruel and wicked,
For that baby could of grown up to of been very clever and gifted,
And if a judgement has been passed that a term of imprisonment shall never be lifted,
For there are those who have tried to have the blame shifted,
And though the years through the system they have changed their names been released struck again moved on and drifted,
And if for a moment my eyes become clouded and misted,
It's just that the journey through life has for many of us has become depressing and very lonely and just a little bit twisted,
And if you think that my spirits have become a little bit placid and somewhat uplifted,
My eyes are tired and sore and just a little bit blistered,
All over my life holistically I have gone through every page, every programme every lane and field and even the moor trying to soothe the child's soul that one day I pray his make shift burial ground could perhaps one day be found and for his tiny body be laid to rest and his spirit with his lord be reunited

And I dream that for all those young and innocent
children that their souls forever someday will once
again be re lighted,
And if any of you one day choose to be
enlightened,
Choose the right path for on your path there is no
need to be frightened.

IF YOU WERE TO WEEP ONE DAY
ONLY IF THE MOUNTAINS BECAME TO
STEEP,
WOULD YOU CRAWL AND WOULD YOU
CREEP,
WOULD YOU SEARCH FOR A LONG LOST
SHEEP,

WHAT IS IT MY FRIEND THAT YOU REALLY
SECRETLY SEEK,
SOMETIMES THE MIND HAS TRAVELLED SO
DEEP,
THAT TO COME OUT IS DANGEROUS EVEN
FOR A PEEK,
THE MIND MIGHT NOT BE STRONG ENOUGH
PSYCHOLOGICALLY WEAK,

THERE ARE TIMES WHEN I DO NOT THINK
BEFORE I SPEAK,
I HAVE SEEN MANY A PERSON SHOUT AND
FREAK,

GARY RUDDICK POEMS

I ALWAYS WANTED TO BE POLISHED LIKE TEAK,
SOME THINGS YOU CAN SEARCH FOR OTHERS YOU DO NOT SEEK,

IF YOU WERE TO SEE ME CURLED UP IN A HEAP,
WOULD YOU ASK YOURSELF AM I NOW OUT OF REACH,
I NEVER CAME HERE FOR AN EDUCATION OR TO TEACH,
I ONLY CAME TO SIT IN THE SUN AND LISTEN TO THE WAVES UPON THE BEACH,

MANY CRIMES I HAVE NEVER COMMITTED,
YET PEOPLE ASK ME TO EDUCATE THEM,
THERE IS THAT SAYING PRACTICE WHAT YOU PREACH,
LIFE'S A BIT LIKE THAT GIANT PEACH,

IM SORRY THAT I ONLY TURNED OUT TO BE A THIEF,
I DREAMED THAT ONE DAY I WOULD GROW UP INTO A CHIEF,
I DIDN'T EXPECT TO BE CAUGHT UP IN ALL THIS GRIEF,
STILL THAT'S SOMETHING I DIDN'T UNDERSTAND AS A CHILD AND THAT WAS MISCHIEF.

Gary Michael Ruddick

GARY RUDDICK POEMS

I'M ONLY WISHING

IF ONLY I COULD TURN BACK THE HANDS OF
TIME, DO YOU EVER THINK WHAT WOULD
OCCUR IFYOU RETURNED TO YESTERDAY,
HOW DO YOU THINK YOUR PATH WOULD
LAY,
DO YOU THINK YOU WOULD BE READING
THIS TODAY,
OR WOULD YOU BE ELSE WHERE EARNING
YOUR PAY,
I GUESS I HAD BETTER BE CAREFUL AS TO
WHAT I SAY,
BUT YOU KNOW ME COME WHAT MAY,
YOU KNOW SERIUOSLY THIS ISNT WHERE I
BELONG OR STAY,
FOR NOW IM JUST LIVING FROM DAY TO DAY,
I DON'T THINK IT MATTERS WHO I AM OR
WHAT I PORTRAY,
I SHALL SAY THIS IS I AM OKAY,
THAT'S BECAUSE FROM A WOMANS ARMS I
HAVE NEVER STRAYED,
YET I AM TROUBLED AND I AM DISMAYED,
BECAUSE FOR MY SOUL THEY TRIED TO
ENSLAVE,
SOME TIMES A SOUL GETS A REPRIEVE,
SOMETIMES AMAN NEEDS TO BREATHE,
THIS ISNT ABOUT WILL YOU OR I GRIEVE,
WILL I OR WONT I OR SHALL I JUST LEAVE,
IF I ASKED YOU FOR A RAZER WOULD I HAVE
TO SAY PLEASE,

WOULD I HAVE TO FALL DOWN UPON MY KNEES,
OR WOULD IT BE EASIER IF I HUNG FROM THE TREES,
EITHER WAY IT WOULD ONLY DISPLEASE,
LEFT ALONE OUTSIDE IN THE FREEZE,
DEATH, WHY DO YOU TEMPT ME, WHY DO YOU TEASE,
TO LEAVE MY LIFE WOULD BE SUCH AN EASE,
AROUND MY NECK THE ROPE WOULD SQEEZE,
SWINGING IN MOTION WITH THE BREEZE,
TOUCHED ONLY BY THE LEAVES,
MOURNED ONLY BY THE HUMMING BEES,
WOULD SUICIDE BE A RELEASE,
WOULD I THERE FIND MY OWN INNER PEACE,
UNBEKNOWN TO ANYONE COULD I WEEP,
FOR THE MOUNTAIN OF LIFE HAS SUDDENLY BECOME TO STEEP,
IF ONE DAY MY BLOOD WERE TO WEEP,
WOULD I JUST BECOME ONE OF THE LOST SHEEP,
ROPES TIED AROUND MY FEET,
JUST ANOTHER SOUL AT THE BOTTOM OF THE HEAP,
SCREAMS SILENCED BY THE HOWL OF THE STORM, WOULD YOU HOLD ME TRY TO KEEP ME WARM,
ARE YOU MY ROSE WITH OUT A THORN,

GARY RUDDICK POEMS

OR ARE YOU CUPIDS TWIN BLOWING HER HORN,
WILL THE SHEPHERDS RETURN AT DAWN,
WOULD THE BEES FLY HIGH IN THEIR SWARM,
I DOUBT IF ANYONE WOULD REALLY MOURN,
JUST ANOTHER CREATURE JUST LIKE A FAWN,
HEART SHREDDED AS IF IT WAS TORN,
WONDERING WHY THE HELL I WAS BORN,
STRANGE WHEN YOU REALISE YOU'RE ONLY A PAWN,
PLAYING TO A CROWD ON THEIR ROYAL LAWN,
HOPING THAT SOON THE GAME WILL END FOR ONLY YOU SENSE THE STORM,
WAITING FOR ANOTHER DAY TO BE REBORN,

Gary Michael Ruddick

IMPACT

Do you know what its like to be on the end of an attack?
When the blood drips and your skin turns black,
Do you know what it's like when your skin is hacked?
Can you imagine when you hit the floor sudden impact?
Do you understand when your body has to burn?
When all you want to do is yearn,
Can you imagine when you are spurned?
When into your heart the stake is turned,
Don't even dream about being placed in ice,
For its like you've been put in a vice,
On your skin the cut of a knife,
To feel the heat isn't very nice,
Can you contemplate being left on your own?
Wondering if its love that you've out grown,
Every thing you do others condone,
No wonder some people only want to be left alone,
If you never had anyone, all because it was something you had done,
You had to change your name so they wouldn't know where you were from,
Where do all those people come from?
Could you imagine the horror if you had been killed by a bomb,
And it was only for your race and really you hadn't done anything wrong,

GARY RUDDICK POEMS

Condemned by the older generation slaughtered by the young,
What has the world gone and done,
Why the hell did man invent the gun?
What went wrong with our savoir our son?
What could have gone wrong?
I no longer understand the hymns or the songs,
I no longer hear theBuddha's gong,
All I hear about is drugs crime and vice,
I suppose it makes you think twice,
I don't understand how some people only have rice,
Who keeps hold of the dice?
Off each other they eat their own rice,
Surely there must be something we could do for them that would be nice,
One day I hope the gods will cut them some slack
, As it seems their always under attack,
Their homes are only that of a shack,
Makes you wonder about impact,

IN MEMORY OF OUR BELOVED FRIEND SMUDGE

To our beloved and best friend,
Who was a very loving and loyal and also
A very faithful companion through the years that
We had the good fortune to share together.
In all of our hearts and memories you will
Always, always be thought of with nothing less than
Love and kindness, joy and happiness
Constantly we reminded of you,
For your gentleness, obedience patience with those
Younger than your self and also for courage and
Strength,
Your ability and awareness as a leader and a
Protector stayed with you to the very end.
Your character and your forever-watchful eyes
And also your silence made you the great dog
That you are and always will be,
You stood out amongst your clan on earth and
We do not doubt our beloved friend that your stature
In heaven shall be that as it were here on earth.
We deeply miss you smudge and we always shall do
For you were more than just a friend you were family.
We are so sad that your journey in life had to end,
You are missed so much our friend.

GARY RUDDICK POEMS

Love from all of us
Rest in peace, dear departed friend.

Gary Michael Ruddick

IN TIME

Have you ever wondered if you were born way
before your time?
Have you thought up, but never committed the
perfect crime,
Have you chased the carrot on the end of the line?
Have you dreamed of finding that perfect gem at
the bottom of the mine?
Have you studied book after book and thought that
perhaps one day you could be equal to Einstein,
Have you looked intensively into yourself and
envisioned that maybe you could be blind,
Surely nature could not be so unkind,
If you keep on searching within your self some
where within a light you will find,
The path that you have passed over you can
never again find,
For events that taken place you can never rewind,
Looking back there are people that you can no
longer find,
For that is the course of the passage of time,
No matter how much you will it time is something
that you cannot rewind,
Though even I will admit I dreamed that I could
through song and rhyme,
For I have delved deep oh so deep into the
darkest caverns of my mind,
Walking through that fragile and unstable blinding
fine line,
Trying to forget the rape and torture of mankind,

GARY RUDDICK POEMS

Trying with every breath and every ounce of
energy to remove myself from this god-forsaken
time,
Screaming in my tortured and tormented soul that
someday no matter I have to climb,
That I shall have to rid myself of all this slime and
man made grime,
Even if I have to return to the beginning of time,
Maybe we could one day all speak the same
language where no one was deaf dumb or blind,
If only nature could have been so kind,
For if only we learnt to understand one another
through one voice through one mind,
Maybe our destiny would not be so blind,
If you look long and hard and deep enough you
just might find,
That somewhere out there is peace for mankind,
Yet we will only find out in time,

I WONDER IF I SHALL EVER BE FREED,
IT NO LONGER MATTERS IF I SHOUT SREAM
OR PLEAD,
FOR FAR TO LONG IVE BEEN PULLED ON A
LEAD,
AT TIMES IVE MADE MYSELF PHYSICALLY
BLEED,
 FOR THAT WAS THE ONLY WAY THAT I
ASSUMED THAT I COULD BE FREED,
SO IT IS TO YOU MY FRIEND THAT I PLEAD,

I DID NOT HAVE A CHOOSE WHEN FROM MY
MOTHER AND FATHER I CAME FROM THEIR
SEED,
I TRIED TO STOP MYSELF BEFORE I WAS
FREED,
YET SOMETHING MAN MADE FORCED ME TO
BREATHE,
NOW ALL I WANT TO DO IS BE AT PEACE AND
LEAVE,
IF I ASKED YOU FOR A REPRIEVE,
I KNOW IN MY MIND YOU WOULD WALK AWAY
AND LEAVE,
THE TEARS THAT I WOULD LEAVE WOULD
NOT BE THOSE THAT COULD BE FREEZED,
FOR THEIR WOULD BE THOSE THAT WOULD
BE PLEASED,
I KNOW FOR SURE MY MIND WOULD BE AT
EASE,
FOR LIFE AND MY LIBERTY HAS ALWAYS
BEEN A TEASE,
YET SOMETHING IN MY MIND FOR A LONG
TIME HAS NEVER BEEN AT EASE,
MY ONLY FRIENDS ARE THESE DAYS ARE
THE BIRDS AND THE BEES
AND MY SINSARE NOW TO HEAVY FOR ME
TO RETURN TO THE TREES,
SO I GET DOWN TO YOU MY FRIEND
UPON MY KNEES,
FOR I AM NOT EVIL NOR AM I A DESEASE,
IN ALL OF MY LIFE   NEVER HAVE IHAD A GOD
BLESS AFTER I SNEEZE,

GARY RUDDICK POEMS

IF I DO MAKE OLD AGE AND I HUFF AND
IPUFF AND I WHEZZ,
THE MOMENTS THAT I HAVE SHARED WITH
YOU WILL NOT BE LOST IN THE BREEZE,
KIND MOMENTS WILL ALWAYS PLEASE,
THESE POEMS ARE A THANKYOU FOR IT'S
VERY RARE THAT I AM AT EASE,
FOR UNBEKNOWN TO YOU I FEEL IN THE
WIND BREEZE,
I JUST HOPE THAT YOU COULD KEEP A
SECRET FOR ME PLEASE,
HERE I AM AGAIN BACK ON MY KNEES,
ANYWAY SWEET DREAMS.GARY RUDDS 4; 16
AM 20 7 2004.

KNOWING

When my blood starts flowing,
My feelings for you start growing

Now that you are knowing,
Will your seeds of love start showing,

If my voice were to become softer and lower
Would your love start to flower?

If the sun once again began to shine,
Would you promise one day to be mine,

If you could you turn back the hands of time,
To be at the beginning of my life line,

Gary Michael Ruddick

If only you could give me a sign
I would willingly turn my back on the life of crime,

If the stars were to give you a path,
Would you open your mind to my craft?

Life wouldn't be sad for we would not want for a
laugh,
I would be your ship and you would be my mast,

In my mind I am the forever knowing,
In my heart for you it is always glowing,

My feelings for you are over flowing,
My light for you will be forever showing,

If you allowed me to cast the light and warmth
over you,
 Then would you know that my love for you is
true?

My colours are that of the purple and blue,
For they are the colours that I offer you,

Mystically spiritually and physically I am in love
with you,
Now I leave the rest up to you,

For I no longer know what to do,

GARY RUDDICK POEMS

All I shall say is that my heart and soul belong to
none other than you,

If you can one day see through my fears,
Please hold on to my tears,

For I look into the mirror and ask are you really
there,
 The eyes look back and ask do you really care,

If you do then show me where,
Please shop me your light and promise that you'll
always be there,

For there are times when I see your spirit floating
in the air,
When you next go please take ME THERE.

Love shall always be magical!
Loves emotions will come in many different kinds
of forms,
It sometimes stays within a person until a child is
born,
Love will even speak to the deaf dumb and the
blind,
They are just as unsure in life even those need
that need help physically and psychologically need
someone to be kind,

Even I have shed many a tear over long forgotten
heartache and pain,

I've been driven to the world of the insane,
Now and again my inner voice tells my I'm not going to be the same,
Yet I ask myself in front of my mirror that the darkness is
Tormenting me with their darkness and their bizarre form of pain,

Once you go through your mind you realise that no one else can see
Your frustration and your inner pain,
For I know it has long been imbedded inside your brain,
Deep down I have emotions that a normal live just wouldn't be the same,
Many of us feel and think like children and that life is just a game,

Love has in this day and age now become some thing of a mystery,
Yet we all have our family and our own family tree,
For now I shall in my heart love and adore you platonically if our needs are to be more than friends then I would love to entwine your body with mine physically,
I would love to entice you with words of love kindness and intimacy,
For I look at you when ever I get the chance to look at you secretly,

GARY RUDDICK POEMS

My thoughts and emotions for you are to me never a mystery,
For the moments I have held you are part of my life and the memories,
Will always be in my heart and soul for now there is little more my love that I need to say,
Only that my feelings for shall now and forever fade away.

Love
Gary
xxxx

MOTHER NATURE

It was a long time ago when Mother Nature was
our maker,
For it was her wisdom and her fertility that created
our nature,
For you only have to look at a man and a woman's
features,
Look at all of our rare and beautiful creatures,
For isn't it our mothers that our really our
protectors and our teachers,
Now long awaited they have become our rightful
preachers,
I feel now that Mother Nature silently is suffering a
deadly internal pain,
For man has laid claim to the blood in her lifeline
which is her vein,
I doubt if forever our earth will continue to take the
strain,
Will Mother Nature ever be the same again?
One day it will be too late for man to take the
blame,
For in my vision life has already been lost to the
insane,
Evolution was not there as a childish game,
Along time ago civilization was kind and tame,
Now nothing and nobody are now the same,
At the end of the day that seriously is a shame,
Are we now just a part of the animal food chain?
The fires underground that endlessly burn to heat
our land,

GARY RUDDICK POEMS

Will a cold and withered hand someday extinguish
them?
Will our children's future be bleak desolate and
damned,
All for the sake of fuel and isn't that down to man/,
Those of you that no longer walk upon the earth
will you be named and shamed,
OR will the whole human race be so deranged
and the land will it be inflamed,
At what stage in time will the different races be
alarmed?
The day that the cattle can no longer be farmed,
Mother Nature how once again can you be loved
and charmed,
Will your precious metals and your exquisite
gems,
Match your beautiful prayers and your sacred
hymns,
Would your pure waters from the heavens cleanse
mankind's sins?
Could the fountains that once were great one day
return in the fresh spring showers?
Nurturing her glorious and exotic flowers,
Will you always and forever be fore ever seeing
and protecting our loved ones and our kin?
For I feel that perhaps that one-day something
may come with the force of the wind,
Who knows mans demise could well begin,
Must we still continue to die for the sake of our
race religion or the colour of our skin?

For I wonder is not your patience starting to grow
thin,
Will the earth continue to nurture the trees and her
fruits those that are there for one and for all,
Will the sun always warm our hearts and our
waters and our soil until the autumn fall?
Shall we once again hear the swans and the
geese passing call?
I ask myself how many of us will one-day fall,
Was our lord really such a fool?
Suppose some of nature's kin were merely used
as tools,

GARY RUDDICK POEMS

MR AND MRS SOCIETY

Mr and Mrs Society do you really understand
what's at stake,
Looking at your society to me it's all so fake,

You try and reform us with you're over powering
will,
You say that we are delusional and that we are ill,

We do not understand the chemicals you make,
We no longer know what we take,

It doesn't matter if it's in a potion or in a pill,
We no longer search for a sensation we no longer
search for a thrill,

How much of yourself do you give or are you just
on the make,
Myself I thought that life was about give and take,

Are you really a professor or just another baker
from the mill?
To be honest the title doesn't matter it's whether
you can fit the bill,

Are you the gardener shifting through the stones
and dirt?
With your sturdy rake,
Are you the birthday child blowing out the candles
on your cake?

Are you the croupier with his magical pack of
cards waiting to break the seal?
Thinking of your commission when you seal the
deal,

Are you the person going to the doctor just for an
ache?
Trying to close your mind to the feeling inside that
it's more than your bones that shake,

Are you the fisherman with his rod and reel?
Sat there with his line and hook waiting for the kill,

Are you now the lifeless body going to his or her
wake?
Will your spirit survive the journey to heaven or will
you break,

Are you the ghost of yesterday and were you ever
real,
Did you come here to haunt and taunt me was that
the devils deal,

Will you honestly ever talk openly with me for do
you really know how to relate?
Or has life passed us all bye and are we now too
late,

GARY RUDDICK POEMS

MY FRIEND

My friend please may I reflect on to you,
For the colour's are more true,
I have already told you about the purple and blue,
Yet I have not told, really expressed how I really fell for you,
It was when I first saw the baby inside of you,
It was then that I fell in love,
For you were more than a brilliant white dove,
For you were from the above,
My heart was filled with your love,
YOU'RE circle of life, 'Love' your rings, a ray of trust shall never rust,
For on your Birthday there shall be I wonder a hush,
Maybe the singing of a thrush,
Could it be the wind in a silent gust,
In my heart & soul I know it's you that I trust,

Love
Gary
X

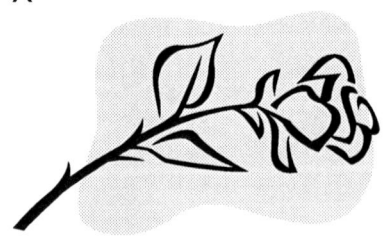

GARY RUDDICK POEMS

MY FUSTRATION

Where do I begin to try to make you understand
that I have my own style or of education,
And if at all possible I shall try to simplify the
meaning of the term elation,
I just hope that you are very patient and that you
do show me a little space and some consideration,
Here I will try and give you a piece of my mind sort
of an evaluation,
Let me catch my breath and I will try my hardest to
give you an explanation,
When the mind and the nervous system reach a
certain level of exhaustion,
The mind and the bodies I think defence system
tries to react in such a way that it causes all kinds
of psychological confusion,
Some of those those are unfortunate to reach the
level of terrible hallucinations,
There are those that I really feel for and they are
those that suffer with term as you are all aware of
and that is the term paranoid delusions,
In my weakness of the mind or possibly my ability
to obtain for the benefit of those trying to
comprehend the functioning of ones mind and the
realization,
That what is taking place today through the
prolonged use of alcohol and the misuse of illegal
and legal substances in our civilization?
Going through in my mind over numerous long
forgotten generations,

GARY RUDDICK POEMS

Somewhere something was forming in the depth of my somewhat elated mind and I was positive that it was not just my imagination,
I have thought many times with my awareness and also with my frustration,
That if those of us unknowingly and apologetically have damaged the cells in which protect and produce a safe guard for our own protection,
 Do you not think that if we are to teach and guide the younger generation?
It is time that that those that are capable of receiving a proper if not higher education,
For is it not you're children that need to be educated about physical and psychological infection,
Would it not be wise for every child to receive physical and psychological inspection?
For who knows what mind boggling boffin will create to induce in the mind of a miner and who knows what it could be a dangerous manifestation,
And a child may never have the chance to reach his graduation,
For he may have accidentally passed away by having an illegal injection,
And my own wayward theory that is a very personal intrusion,
So there isn't any more that I can explain concerning the state of our nation,
And I think I hope that by reading this you may also if possible be able to understand and comprehend the phrase word association,

If those that are capable of creating a natural form of mood stabilizer then I may be persuaded to take up medicine but only for the fascination,
But to tell the truth I haven't got the patience to learn an education,
If you put your mind to it and your imagination,
In time you could eventually produce spiritually and physically you own precious beautiful creation,
Do not think ill of me if I send myself accidentally into the depths of damnation,
For I do not agree to the thoughts of self mutation,
So to be on the safe side for you my friend I shall endure the process of taking some form of medication,

GARY RUDDICK POEMS

MY LITTLE FEATHERED FRIEND

I write this to you to make amends,
To all of my little feathered friends,
There are those that say to hunt a bird is part of a trend,
Some things I do not comprehend,

Strange how we all enjoy the egg,
Yet it is man that is the one that has to beg,
My little friends, do you think I'm pulling your leg,
They dip the yoke with their bread,

They cook the chicken for the leg and breast,
Isn't it time they gave the bird a rest,
For on earth even man is only a guest,
This day and age they're more than a pest,

This isn't a final request,
I guess its kind of a test,
But do you have to steal the eggs out of her nest,
For it is not only the child on earth that is blest,

Man will never advance for the animal kingdom has not been enhanced,
Spiritual figures have worn many feathers and danced,
Too many people have taken a chance,
Yet they still-hunt the bird that sits waiting patiently on the branch,

Gary Michael Ruddick

The colours that you represent in your feathers,
Will protect you in all weathers,
Some of you wear colours on your leathers,
Yet how many wear the colour of the heather,

Your tools are that of your claws,
They have protected you through many wars,
In your time you have opened many doors,
Man does not think to stop or pause,

Man even names his woman after a bird,
Is that an after thought as to me that is absurd?
Do they not know the passage or passion even of
words?
They even demean you my precious birds,

Even to you my little beautiful thrush,
Who has the softness of a brush?
They name you in the form of a disease as in
thrush,
No wonder when they die their bodies turn in the
earth to slush,

Even the black and white magpies of the sky they
call you a thief.
Little do they know you are of the stature of a
chief?
So what if you cause a little bit of mischief,
Your call is that of peace,

Nature has dreamed you fit for the skies,

GARY RUDDICK POEMS

For I see the love for freedom that you hold in your
eyes,
Man shall never learn where you all go when you
die,
No matter what they try for man shall be denied,

They think they know how you glide,
Yet a bird is not a plane so they do not collide,
They do not know the spirit inside,
For the bird never had the chance to live or die,

Exotic birds are kept locked in a cage,
Inside the birds are filled with a rage,
Yet they have the calmness of the ancient sage,
Some stories do not continue into another page,

You think they sit there in a daze.
They have watched and listened through every
age,
They sit and watch the sunrays,
Counting the silent days,

They watch who comes and who stays,
You think they sit around and laze,
They live their lives in smoke and haze,
Yet no one sees them into the grave,

They hunt only nature,
For it is the food of their maker,
Only they know their maker,

Gary Michael Ruddick

For it is not the end when you meet the undertaker,

There are many statures in the bird society,
There are all kinds of varieties,
Most have a meaning and all are niceties,
For in my world they all sing to me,

Some sing with the voice of a harp.
Some have teeth as sharp as a sharp,
None of them belong to the dark,
Their home long ago was that of the ark,

A vessel that was made of wood,
For nature was given another chance to see if it was good,
Against time the bird has stood,
Yet would you protect a magpie if you could?

For there are those that do good,
Well they would if they could,
Yet most of nature is misunderstood,
That is why they live in the woods,

Even the merry men wore brown and greens,
They learned to become thieves,
 They lived among the bush and the trees,
Nature was meant for all creatures to be free,

Have you wondered about the god pan?
He lived for the birds and of course man.

GARY RUDDICK POEMS

Yet the leaves are wrote upon every creatures hand,
That is something I doubt you will ever understand, Gary Ruddick.

MY WORLD IN VIEW WITHOUT YOU

There are times when I see beyond just a picture,
Looking into you I wonder who's with you,
In my mind you are a permanent fixture,
Are you really this stunning and are you really true,

I call your name as you float by in the wind,
I ask myself could I one day join you in the wind,
I do not know where to look for you for there are times when I am blind,
Your voice and your light guides me gently so I know that you're not unkind,

I do wish we could travel back to the beginning of time,
When I was yours and you were my mine,
The mountains wouldn't have been so hard to climb,
I would not have chosen the life of crime,

Sometimes it's easier to put things down in the form of a rhyme,
Than catch a fish at the end of a line,
Or kill a man hidden by a secret mine,
Looking for his body never a piece of him would you find?

Looking into the blue and grey sky line,
I see some friends fly by yours and mine,

GARY RUDDICK POEMS

I guess it's time to feed them as it's dinner time,
Once these have eaten they'll be fine,

Funny little thing these creatures of our time,
When they talk the sun does shine,
If only I could turn back the hands of time,
For all I ask is that once if only once you put your hand in mine,

For a more genuine tender love you could never hope to find,
I hope some day my path you find,
I just pray that you to have not become blind,
To the ways of the beast of so called mankind,

In my heart and soul I always shall be tender and kind,
For up above I am one of a kind,
There are others of their own kind,
But some of us stem from the ancient time.

      Sincerely yours
      Gary Michael Ruddick.

Gary Michael Ruddick

ONCE I WAS A SOLDIER

Along time from here I declared that from that day
I had chosen to walk my path alone,
For my heart had been broken and until now it
was as cold and as hard as stone,
You must never break the spirit of a man for it is
much stronger than the bone,
And if you try I ask that you do not for it is some
thing, which I deeply condone.

As of yet I have not taken a life with these pair of
hands,
My spirit has already flown far out across the
lands,
My footprints are the only trace that I have walked
onto the sands,
Long before you heard my name I had already
made my plans,

Only once in my life have I picked up arms against
a man,
And it was unto my self that I left a long and deep
brand,
For it was on that day that I vowed for any child to
take a stand,
And if I had chosen not to forever in hell I would
have been damned.

For what reason do you try to gain entry past a
mans defence,

GARY RUDDICK POEMS

If it was at the cost of his life would it honestly
been worth the expense,
To see his body cold and motionless lay out in a
trench,
Surely it is not worth to learn of his long forgotten
experience.

For if one day the you open the pages and reveal
the secrets of your folder,
It may not be at present for it may come about
when he is much older,
And if that time should ever arise would you let
him cry on your shoulder,
Just remember though his heart just may have
grown colder.

All through his life he has stared at a blank page,
He got confused, lost in past thoughts, ended up
in a rage,
He always dreamed that one day he would write
for the stage,
He knows now that tomorrow has been and gone
and he has come of age.

He looks back over distant events and everything
to him now is just a haze,
Drinking and taking drugs that was to him only a
crave,
Strange when you look back on your life to come
back to the present is a bit like entering a maze,

Thank goodness it's not to far away until I can sit back and enjoy reaching my old age.

GARY RUDDICK POEMS

ONLY FOR YOU MY FRIEND

Without you long ago I would have died,
Emotions have been released deep down inside,
The times that I have broken down and cried,
Only you were close by my side,

Looking back at those difficult years,
I ask you why am I still here,
With you I have never had anything to fear,
All I ask is that you remain quite near,

In your presence I am always filled with a very
deep emotion,
I dream that you would one day accept my love
and devotion,
My soul tells me that you are the purest woman in
all of creation,
To me it its you that has become more than a
revelation,

In my dreams I wonder if it is you whispering
softly: what will be will be...
Taking me to the heavens secretly protecting and
loving me,
Freeing my tormented soul for all of eternity,
Removing the pain that has always dwelled inside
of me,

Only in your presence can I find the thoughts for
reflection,

Holding my breath if you choose to look in my direction,
Looking into your eyes I know your given me a psychological examination,
In my mind no one else could ever have such a high education,

In time you have become much more than a friend,
Some times there are moments that I pray that it shall never end,
It's something that I have not wanted to comprehend,
The thoughts of never holding you close are that ill fall from grace and I cant pretend,

I shift through my emotions day and night,
Searching for your presence at the first light,
Shadows overwhelm me and within myself I begin once more to fight,
Drifting in and out of reality your gentle voice brings me out of the dark and into the light,

All my life I have remained quiet and afraid to speak,
In your presence once more I am that child again innocent and weak,
Longing for love and affection is that to much for a child to seek,
Insecure am I just another lost and lonely freak,

GARY RUDDICK POEMS

I realise that my love for you has long ago been denied,
Another love poem never to be replied,
Over the years I have now lost count of how many tears for you I have cried,
The love I shall always carry for you could never have died,

No one could ever take the emotions that for you are embedded deep inside,
For you gave me something back and that is my pride, love Gary xx

Gary Michael Ruddick

PLAYING THE GAME

Trying to pretend that I am crazy and insane,
Playing out delusions as in the story of life we are
all actors and life is just a game,
Chemicals flowing freely around my body and my
brain,
Watching eyes that may hide a deep imbedded
shame,
Wondering if whom you call yourself is your proper
first or your marriage name,
Thinking to myself that the majority have become
shadows of their former self and their minds have
now become lame,
Within my self I feel a sense of satisfaction for my
spirit you cannot contain,
Looking at man it seems the system and the drugs
have physically and psychologically made them
silent and submissive and tame,
Myself I am not just into the aggression or that
volatile game,
For my sense of self-conviction is something I do
not want connected to my name,
I do have fleeting moments, only brief though that
I remember times of pain,
Yet if I recalled every emotion that I have felt then
I may enter the path of the insane,
Yet my self-preservation and my intuition make
me think and consciously refrain,

GARY RUDDICK POEMS

For I have ventured down that path of life and I forbid myself to walk down that self-defeating path again,

My misfortune that for now I have to preserve until my liberty I shall one day regain,

My past is not one of shame,

For I do not have those feelings of remorse in the spheres of my brain,

My psychological thinking since I arrived here has due to my self preservation somewhat changed,

I can assure those that think that they know the workings of my brain,

That my thoughts and experiences are not of an individual, who through experiences through narcotics has now become deranged,

For I feel that your assessments of my past and present situations have to you

Must seem somewhat strange,

Yet do you understand how the light and the dark forces intermingle confer silently and in secret thoughts telepathically exchange,

My spiritual light shall guide you and that my friend s shall never change.

REMEMBERING YOUR NAME

Shifting through the years trying to remember your name,
Wondering if you still look the same,
Recalling your smile that always graced your face,
Even to this day I doubt if it would be out of place,
Remembering the softness in your voice,
How could I not love you my heart gave me no choice,
Remembering the colour of the sky in the light of your eyes,
Looking deep within them I realised that you were kind intelligent and wise,
Remembering the moments with you that I felt true desire,
The love I felt then and do to this day warms my heart and soul like a burning fire,
Remembering how you used to hold yourself and the way you used to dress,
Your beauty always astonished me and every time I saw you I had to catch my breath,
Remembering the colour the cut and tone of your hair,
Recalling your gentle approach realising from the moment I first saw you that you really do care,
You were always understanding, honest, gentle, kind and fair.
Looking back on those times I really needed a friend so thank you for being there,

GARY RUDDICK POEMS

Remembering how I always dreamed that maybe
one day I might hold you in my arms,
Wishing that perhaps I could somehow gain your
love and trust with my charms,
Remembering that once you told me that beauty
had to come from within,
For a moment I can remember the softness and
paleness of your skin,
The figure of you in a dress I shall carry in my
mind until I die,
I still fantasies to this day of kissing the softness of
the inside your thigh,
Remembering your figure desperately once again
I let out a long lost sigh,
The picture of you in my soul will stay with me
long after I have died,
I could never have stopped loving even if I had of
tried,
My only regret was that for all of my poems and
letters not once have you replied,
Many years now have passed and gone by,
Many long nights I have lain here alone and cried,
Wishing that I would wake one day to find you
asleep by my side,
In my dreams I have willed it, believe me I have
tried,
If only the heavens could one day be defied,
Come to think of it, how could I forget your name?
If I did I would only have myself to blame,
Strange how love can make you insane,
Amanda was your lovely name.

Gary Michael Ruddick

Love
Gary
 X

SAMHAIN

IN THIS TIME OF THE YEAR THERE IS NO
TIME OF FEAR,
FOR THERE ARE RITUALS THAT ARE
RELIGIOUSLY PERFORMED BY GODS AND
GODDESSES ALL THRUOGH THE YEAR,
THERE IS MUCH LAUGHTER WINE FOOD AND
CHEER,
THE LIVING AND THE DEAD ALL GATHER
HERE,
EVERY SOUL THAT HAS SINCE TIME BEGUN
HAS PASSED THROUGH HERE,
HIGH PRIESTS AND PRIESTESS PRAY TO THE
FORCES OF THE DARK AND TO THE LIGHT,
EVOKING SPIRITS THAT FOR CENTURIES
HAVE REMAINED SILENT UNTIL THE TIME
WAS RIGHT,
FIRES ARE BURNING LONG INTO THE COLD
WINTERS NIGHT,
CHILDREN SHADOWS WARMING
THEMSELVES BY THE FIRE THEIR LAUGHTER
ECHOING INTO THE NIGHT,
RITUALS OF FIRST SECOND AND THIRD
DEGREE INITIATONS,
RUNES BEING SPOKEN FROM A SACRED AND
LONG LOST RELIGION,
WITCHES WEARING THEIR TRADITIONAL
DRESS OF ATTIRE,
INCENSES FROM AROUND THE WORLD
BEING SPINKLED UNTO THE FIRE,

LANTERNS PLACED IN THE NORTH EAST
WEST AND SOUTH,
RUNES BEING SPOKEN IN DIFFERENT
TONGUES FROM THEIR MOUTH,
CAULDRONS FILLED WITH ALL SECRET
RECIPIES OF HERBS AND PLANTS,
CHILDREN SINGING AND DANCING WITCHES
PRAYING IN A SACRED CHANT,
KINGS AND QUEENS COMING TOGETHER
UNITED IN PEACE LAYING DOWN THEIR
ATHAMES AND THEIR SWORD,
A FEMALE SINGS AS MUSIC SEEMS TO ECHO
FROM THE MOON,
SPIRITS OF THE DEAD AND THOSE LIVING
SEEM TO BE DANCING TO A MAGICAL TUNE,
SPELLS HAVE BEEN CASTE UPON EVERY
NATION UPON THE EARTH,
EVERY DRUID SORCERESS HEALERS
WIZARDS THAT DWELL IN THE LAND ARE
TONIGHT TRYING TO REMOVE A CURSE,
GOBLINS ELVES FAIRIES AND ALL THE
MYSTICS IN THE LAND,
ARE READING THE PATHS ON THEIR
CHILDRENS HAND,
TAROT CARDS ARE BEING DEALT FASTER
THAN THE WINDS CAN REMOVE THE
FOOTPRINTS IN THE SAND,
GODS AND GODDESES HAVE SAID CAN I
REMOVE THE BLOOD SPILLED ACROSS THE
LAND,

GARY RUDDICK POEMS

FOR THE INNOCENT HAVE BEEN FORSAKEN
AND SOME OF US FEEL THEY ARE DAMNED,
TO ME IT SEEMS THAT EVERY CHILD FOR
SOME REASON HAS THEIR OWN BRAND,
I ASK YOU WHY IS DEATH IN SUCH A HIGH
DEMAND,
THE CAULDONS ARE READY THE BROTH AND
THE BREAD HAS COOLED DOWN,
TONIGHT IS THE SACRED SABBAT AND
EVERY CHILD SHALL BE GIVEN A CROWN,
FOR THE STONES IN HENGE HAVE BEEN
PLACED IN THE GROUND, THE INNOCENT
SLEEP PEACEFULLY NOT MAKING A SOUND

SLEEP DEPREVATION

Watching the night turn into the day with a certain
amount of anticipation,
Trying to focus on your words of concern yet the
tiredness has taken hold and vie lost my thought
of concentration,
Thinking that I could survive without any sleep,
music and telly my only form of relaxation,
Days and nights gone by all I sense now is
confusion,
Looking at the walls wondering is this all part of a
self induced hallucination, it seems as if my reality
has turned into a nightmare and you're really the
devil and in my mind you're real so I guess your
human,
Looking into the mirror I see only myself so it has
to be a delusion,
Turning on the radio I can pick up on any secret
message it's a magical way of communication,
No one knows I understand that's its why it has its
weird kind of fascination,
Your mind pleading for sleep yet you search for a
higher elation,
All sensibility long gone as you on the verge of
exhaustion,
Everyone telling you to rest yet you take no heed
of his or her caution,
Your mind is awake yet your body now is moving
in slow motion,
Every sound seems like an explosion,

GARY RUDDICK POEMS

Everybody seems to making some sort of commotion,

People pleading with you to take some form of light sedation,

In your mind you think that every thing you read is a revelation,

For others you lose touch with their feelings and you have no consideration,

Desperately those that care urges you to take a higher do of medication,

Silently you reach the point where all you sense is frustration,

For in your deluded mind their all pointing the finger and you wait in disbelief and anticipation,

Waiting for the next song to further your muddled education,

Thinking coffee and tea will help you beat off this sleep deprivation,

Looking for the natural high this time you're searching for a natural spiritual elevation,

For far too long you have been held down and force-fed intramuscular medication,

It runs through your body and feels like corrosion,

They say they care and it's their way of devotion,

As long as they get paid for giving you some form of pill or potion,

You are now void of any form of feelings or emotion,

Funny how if some of you stood up and spoke your mind you would not find yourself in certain situation,

The frame of mind I'm in today is not due to care and medication,
It comes down my own self-satisfaction,
I only wish you had the same kind of education,
Instead of your text book illustration,
Another poem for cross-examination,
It's deeper with you though professor as it's a verbal conversation,
Who knows with your pen and paper you may one day change the mental health for the future generation,
I just hope you don't get confused and suffer any form of sleep deprivation,
As it's not a very nice sensation,
And that's the truth it's a first class education its all to with self-preservation.

GARY RUDDICK POEMS

STILL DREAMING

LOOKING INTO THE SHADOWS OF YOUR
OWN MIND,
HAVE YOU WONDERED JUST WHAT YOU
MIGHT FIND,
PLEASE BELIEVE ME FOR I AM NOT BLIND,
BUT SOME MOUNTAINS WERE NEVER
MEANT TO BE CLIMBED,

FOR YOU DO NOT KNOW WHAT TO EXPECT
OR WHAT YOU MAY FIND,
THERE IS MORE TO US THAN JUST THE PATH
OF MANKIND
YOU DO NOT HAVE TO HAVE THE MIND OF
EINSTIEN,
TO GO BACK INTO HISTORY OR THAT
CHOSEN BY THE BLIND

SINCE THE BEGINNING OF TIME MAN NEVER
KNEW THE RHYME,
SO AS THE DAYS AND NIGHTS COMBINED,
I DECIDED TO MAKE UP SOME OF MINE,
FOR WE ALL MUST COME FROM ONE TREE
OR ANOTHER AND I COME FROM A VINE,

FOR IF YOU WERE TO DRINK FROM ME I AM
THE SWEETEST OF WINE,
BUT NOT HERE MAYBE IN ANOTHER TIME,
ONE OR TWO WOMAN HAVE HAD THE
PLEASURE BUT THEIR FAR FROM MY MIND,

I HAVE ONLY FONDEST THOUGHTS OF THEM
FOR THEY WERE KIND

SOMETIMES I DREAM THAT SOMEDAY YOU
COULD BE MINE,
TURNING THE CLOCK HANDS BACK ON TIME,
THAT TO ME WOULD BE THE PERFECT
CRIME,
BRINGING YOU BACK TO YOUR YOUTH AND
BEAUTY LISTENING TO THE CHURCH BELLS
CHIME,

YESTERDAYS GONE NOW SO I GUESS YOUR
BLIND,
I DOUBT IF YOU THINK OF ME IN YOUR MIND,
I MUST BE OUT OF SINZH AND OUT OF TIME,
THE PROGRESS OF THE MIND YOU CANT
REWIND,

BUT DON'T CONCERN YOURSELF ABOUT ME
ILL BE FINE,
ANOTHER LIFE ILL BE YOURS AND YOULL BE
MINE,
THAT'S IF YOU'RE PREPARED TO COME
ACROSS ONTO MY LINE,
MY LOVE I SHALL NOT WAIT UNTIL THE END
OF TIME,

ARE NAMES ARE INBEDDED IN FINE LINE,
MY HAND IN YOURS AND YOURS IN MINE,

GARY RUDDICK POEMS

I DREAMED AS A CHILD THE MOUNTAINS
TOGETHER WE WOULD CLIMD,
FOR OUR BLOODLINE SHALL NOW AND
FOREVER NEVER BE IN DECLINE,

OUR CHIDREN OUR IN OUR OWN UNIQUE
DESIGN,
LOVE IN THE HEART ALWAYS HAS STAYED
THE TEST OF TIME,
AS THEIR FATHER I COULD NEVER RESIGN,
SO GIVE THEM TIME FOR THEY BOTH
ONEDAY SHALL SHINE,
LOVE
GARY MICHAEL RUDDICK

Stream lining visions of the past present and
future,
Are we just another form of creature?
Don't tell me imp destined to be a futuristic
feature,
For my best side isn't that in a picture,
For vie already drank the brew they made in their
mixture,
So my mind body and soul are here as a
permanent fixture,
You have never touched me and I am of the
softest texture,
Would you like to come with me on a beautiful
adventure?
The day's week's month's years would not count
on your usual calendar,

Gary Michael Ruddick

It wouldn't matter if you were born between the month of January or December,
For once long ago there were thirteen as you made me remember,
Never have I been so deep in to a number,
 But I was born a time before the summer,
Very rarely do I fall into a slumber,
If ever I do it's because of the weather,
Or it's because your skin is scented in lavender,
Strange vie never seen you under the weather,
Yet your soul flits into your eyes the colour of heather,
That is how my dear friend I know you're clever,
I shall always have fond memories of you forever and ever,
And in your mind I hear you saying yes Gary whatever,

GARY RUDDICK POEMS

ALL IN GOOD TIME

The path that I have already walked on is none
other than mine,
For if you choose to follow you could quite easily
lose your mind,
For if you keep on searching into the past and
therefore you could become blind,
The reason I say this is to return to yesterday
would be very hard to find,
So as of today I can no longer think back for it
takes up too much of my present time,
So for a little piece of time I choose to remain
silent and just relax and unwind,
I guess I can tell you that I really am fine,
There are some things in life that have occurred
that no matter what you say or do, you could
never unwind,
Some things stay with you and some things you
leave behind,
The quote is: "the blind shall lead the blind"
For it i8 the deaf, dumb and blind that we need to
be kind, so please be patient with those less
fortunate than you if you do not mind,
For they do not see the wording of the rhyme,
Also they do not understand or hear the beat of
the music playing in time,
There are those that have no voice and no sound
to read speak or sing the next line,
I ask you why nature does to those children such
an injustice for surely your way out of line,

For in my eyes you have committed an unforgivable crime,
I thought that man and woman were your perfect design,
Look into the souls that have lost their way and are in darkness and torment and are in a bottomless mine,
For you cannot see even with a light into the caverns of their mind,
Yet you perceiver with your understanding comforting presence
At a distance which in many a fraternity you could never again ever hope to find,
In my time here you have been almost like family and you have always given me your precious time,
And that really makes me wonder why you are doctors and nurses so polite and so kind,
As when we come to you all covered in dirt and grime,
And when we speak, some of us are way out of line,
Spitting and snarling as if you were slime,
Please be patient for some have been locked up for a very long time,
In my time I've often wondered if we all know that friendly hand sign,
And if I decided for all time to retire from the life of crime,
We all know that nobody and I mean nobody can turn back the hands of time,

GARY RUDDICK POEMS

If there was a moment in my life that I felt that I could not continue to rhyme,

I would without a moment's doubt I would lay down my life and end my bloodline,

Yet day after day you always come up to me just in the moment of time,

And it's always the same little pleasant one line,

Gary, how are you feeling today? And I always say, I'm fine,

For the moment ill briefly put down my pen and resign,

If I offered you my love platonically and held out my hand as an offering and a bond of friend ship would you take hold of mine,

For my journey to this day through life has been blind,

And if it wasn't for your company and laughter the truth is I would of without a doubt lost my mind,

So this is a special thank you, all of you for looking after the likes of me, thank you for being so kind,

In my heart if I could and I would give you all an award as a whole, for I feel that you are the strength and you have the knowledge that keeps our country and if not the world and your fraternity is I guess the foundations of mankind,

And the truth is: are we all one of a kind?

Yours sincerely.

GARY.

Gary Michael Ruddick

THE SECRET CIRCLE OF THIRTEEN OLD ONES.

I AM THE FIRST OF THEOLD ONES.I HAVE SEEN THEDAWN OF TIME, FROM THE SUNS BEYOND ARE EARTH.MEN CALL ME THETHE STONE GODDESS, OLD, STEADFAST, AND WISE,

I AM THE SECOND OF THE OLD ONES.I OPENED MY ARMS TO THE FIRST ONE, AND COOLED HER FIRE WITH MY BREATH.I WAS THE PRI ORDIAL MOVEMENT, THE FIRST STIRRING OF THE WINDS.MEN CALL ME THE FATHER OF CHAOS.

I AM THE THIRD OF THE OLD ONES.I WAS THE WATERS UPON THE FACE OF THE TWO. FROM MYDEPTH ALL LIFE WAS FORMED.MY FACE WAS SOFTENED BY THE BREATH OF THE SECOND ONE.MEN CALL ME MARA, THE BITTER ONE, THE SEA

I AM THE FOURTH OF THE OLD ONES. GAVE MY WARMTH TO THE THREE.FROM MY BRILLIANCETHE THIRD ONE WAS GIVEN BEAUTY.MEN AND WOMAN CALL ME SOL, THE SUN.

I AM THE FIFTH OF THE OLD ONES.I GAVE MY LIGHT TO THE DARKNESS.MINE ARE THE TIDES TO RULE.THOUGH MY BROTHER THE FOURTH SHOWS GREATER BRILLIANCE, I TOO HAVE BEAUTY. MEN CALL ME THE VIRGIN, ALSO I AM NAMED LUNA, THE MOON.

I AM SIXTH OF THE OLD ONES.I RIDE THE EARTH ON CLOVEN FEET, OR ON WINGS OF AIR. I AM THE HUNTER AND THE HUNTED.STAG AND HORSE, BIRD AND BEAST ARE MINE, AND WITH THE AID OF THE FIFTH, WHOSE CALL MUST ANSWER, I REPRODUCE MY OWN KIND. MEN AND WOMAN KIL IN LUST FOR ME.I AM NAMED HERNE OR PAN, CERNUNNOS OR THE HORNED ONE.

I AM SEVENTH OF THE OLD ONES.I AM THE FLORAL ONE, ALL LAUGHTER AND JOY ARE MINE/ WITH THE SIXTH; I CALL ALL LIVING THINGS TO JOIN IN OUR MAGICAL DANCE. I AM THE ETERNAL HE AND SHE WHO KNOWS NOT DESTRUCTION. THE SILVER FISH ARE MINE, AS ARE THE SPINNERS OF SILKEN WEBS, THE WEAVERS OF DREAMS.MEN KNOW ME AS THEIR FATHER AND MOTHER, AND CALL ME GREAT.

I AM THE EIGHTH OF THE OLD ONES.I AM A MYSTERY, FOR I AM MY OWN TWIN.MY TWO FACED ARE LIFE AND LIGHT.SOL AND THE WINDS THAT COOL HIM ARE BOTH OF MY ESSENCE. MEN AND WOMAN KNOW ME AS THE MOVER AND THE FERTILISER, CALL ME AIR AND FIRE.

I AM THE NINTH OF THE OLD ONES.WITH THE EIGHTH, I AM WHOLENESS, FOR I AM LOVE AND LAW.THE FATHER OF CHAOSTHE BITTER SEA ARE MY PARENTS.MEN AND WOMAN KNOW ME AS THENOURISER ANDAND SHAPE

GIVER, AND CALL ME WATER AND EARTH.MY
BROTHER THE EIGHTH AND I ARE THE
QUARTERED CIRCLE OF CREATION.

I AM THE TENTH OF THE OLD ONES. I AM THE
PUPIL OF ALL THE OTHERS.I BEGIN WITH
FOUR, AND THEN HAVE TWO, AND END WITH
THREE. FROM THE BELLY I CAME, AND TO
THE WOMB I GO.I AM NOTHING AND YET I AM
LORD OF ALL.I SHALL CEASE, AND YET
RETURN. I AM GOOD, YET I AM MORE
TERRIBLE THAN THOSE WHO HAVE GONE
BEFORE. I AM MAN.

I AM THE ELEVENTH OF THE OLD ONES.I TOO
AM THE PUPIL. WITH THE TENTH I SEEK THE
TRUTH. THERE IS NO HE WITHOUT SHE.MINE
IS THE GREAT CAULDRON OF CREATION,
YET AM I EVER VIRGIN.I AM EVEN MORE
TERRIBLE THAT THE TENTH, FOR LOGIC AND
REASON ARE NOT MINE WHEN MY LITTLE
ONES ARE DESTROYED BY ANY OF THE
OTHERS.I AMWARM YET COLD, GENTLE YET
DESTRUCTIVE .I MIRROR THE STONE ONE
AND THE FLORAL ONE.I AM WOMAN.

I AM THE TWELFTH OF THE OLD ONES.HIDE
FROM MY FACE IF YOU WILL, BUT KNOW
THAT I AM THE MOST POWERFUL OF ALL.THE
TENTH AND ELEVENTH DANCE WITH ME, AND
EVEN THE FLORAL ONE WEEPS SUMMER
TEARS AT MY COMMAND.FOR I AM AN EVER
TURNING WHEEL.I AM THE SPINNER AND THE
WEAVER, AND ALSO I CUT THE SILVER SILK

CORDS OF TIME.MEN AND WOMAN KNOW ME AS FATE, AND I AM THE HERMAPHRODITE, I AM THE THIRTEENTH OF THE OLD ONES.I AM THE SHADOW OF THE SANCTUARY, AND THE SILVER WHEEL OF ARIANHOOD.I AM FEARED, YET LOVED AND OFTEN YEARNED FOR.I RIDE MY WHITE MARE OVER THE BATTLEFIELDS, AND IN MY ARMS THE SICK AND TIRED FIND REST.WE SHALL BE TOGETHER MANY TIMES, FOR THOUGH I AM THE VICTOR, YET AM I ALSO THE LONLIEST OF ALL THE THIRTEEN.TO SEEK THE TWELVE IS TO KNOW THAT I AM BUT AN ILLUSION.WOE IS TO ME THE THIRTEENTH ONE-AND YET ALL JOY IS MINE ALSO, FOR FROMMY EMBRACE IS RENEWED LIFE, AND TO KNOW ME IS TO MEET,KNOW, REMEMBER, AND TO LOVE AGAIN.MEN AND WOMAN KNOW ME AS DEATH-YET I AM THE COMFORTER AND RENEWER, THE CORRECTING PRINCIPLE IN CREATION. THE SCYTHE AND THE VICTORS CROWN ARE MINE, FOR ALL THE THIRTEEN, I AM THE ONLY ONE WHOS LIGHT SHALL BURN FOR ETERNITY, FOR I AM THE SACRED PATH FOR THOSE THAT HAVE GONE BEFORE, THOSE THAT ARE PRESENT AND FOR THOSE THAT ARE YET TO COME .I AM THE MYSTERIES OF TIME PAST AND MYSTERIES THAT MAN AND WOMAN HAVE YET TO FIND ON THEIR JOURNEY THROUGH LIFE, WITH THE WITH

GARY RUDDICK POEMS

THE DARKNES OF THE SILENT NIGHT THEIR SHADOWS SILLETTOED BY THE LIGHT OF THE MOON.OR GOVERNED BY FIRE OF THE SUN ON A WARM SUMMERS DAY, MY SPIRIT TRAVELS UPON THE WIND GENTLY AT TIMES BOWING THE FLOWERS IN MY PASSING, OR IF MY TEARS ARE HEAVY THEN THEY SHALL BLOW FORTH AT SUCH A SPEED AND WITH SUCH FORCE, THAT EVEN THE CURRENTS OF THE DEEPEST OCEAN SHALL TWIST AND TURN THAT EVERY FISH SHALL BE THROWN UPON THE LAND.MY VOICE WIL BE THAT OF A CHILD WHEN I AM LOVED AND WHEN I CAN RETURN MY LOVE TO YOU,YET IF I AM ANGRY MY THUNDER SHALL ROAR AND MOUNTAINS SHALL CRUMBLE AND BECOME DUST . MY LIGHT IS EQUAL IN THE DAY AND IN THE NIGHT FOR MY STRIKE IS FROM THE HEAVENS AND NO MORTAL COULD EVER WITHSTAND MY MIGHT, YET IN SUMMER I AM THE ANGELS DELIGHT, FOR THEY KNOW ME FOR THEY SEE ME AT FIRST LIGHT,
AT NIGHT I AM THE SHEPHARD FOR THAT IS MY TRUE COLOUR.
 THE PATH YOU ALL CHOSE TO TAKE SHALL ALWAYS BE YOUR OWN,
 FOR THERE ARE MANY COLOURS IN THE RAINBOW YET ONLY MINE HAS A ROYAL THRONE, YET MY CHILDREN IF YOU GET LOST CALL ON ME YOUR TRUE FRIEND AND I SHALL BRING YOU ALL HOME. GARY XX

Gary Michael Ruddick

GARY RUDDICK POEMS

THE STARS ARE A PASSAGE PAST THE
MOON,
STRANGE HOW ALL MANS PREDICTIONS
WERE PREDICTED TO SOON,
NO, ONE REALLY KNOWS THE POWER OF
THE MOON,
THE SWELL OF THE WATERS SHALL ONCE
AGAIN BRING A NOTHER MONSOON,
FLOODS WILL RISE AS NUCLEAR ROCKETS
UNDER WATER ONCE AGAIN SILENTLY GO
BOOM,

NEVER AGAIN SHALL NEPTUNE BECOME
ANOTHER GROOM,
FOR A GODDESS HAS CHANGED HER LIGHT
FOR THE SWISH OF A BROOM,
SEALING IN THE EARTH FOR ALL ETENITY IN
THE DARK AND THE GLOOM,
EVERY MAN WOMAN AND CHILD ARE
DESTINED FOR A TOMB,

DID YOU HONESTLY THINK THAT YOU COULD
FEED ME DRUGS IN A NEEDLE OR FOOD
FROM A SPOON,
WERE YOU SERIOUS THAT YOU COULD KEEP
ME WARM WITH A SOFT BLANKET MADE
FROM A LOOM,
THE LIGHT YOU ONCE POSSESED HAS NOW
TURNED TO GLOOM
DID YOU THINK THAT I WAS BORN UNDER A
MUSHROOM,

YOUR PRESENCE COULD NEVER HAVE MADE
ME BLOOM,
FOR MY LIGHT WAS TAKEN AWAY ALL TO
SOON
SO ALONE I SHALL ENTER MY TOMB,
FOR IN MY MIND YOU HAVE NO ROOM

THE DARK HERE ON EARTH SHALL FOREVER
LOOM,
FOR MOTHER NATURE SEALED HER OWN
TOMB,
THERE WAS ONCE UPON A TIME A MOMENT
THAT I THOUGHT YOU MIGHT FLOWER AND
BLOOM,

EVOLUTION AND NATURE WERE CREATED
TO SOON,
MAN SLAUGHTERED THE WHALE AND THE
SEAL WITH A HOOK AND HARPOON,
THE HEAVENS LIGHTS ARE NOW SILENT AND
DARK AND NOT A MOMENT TO SOON,
EVEN YOUR CANDLES WILL NOT SHOW THE
SHADOWS WAITING SILENTLY IN THE ROOM.

IF YOU THINK YOU KNOW THE POWER OF
THE RUNE,
FOR IT IS NOT AN ANGELS HARP THAT PLAYS
MY TUNE,
FOR DEATH IS YOUR DEPARTURE...THAT
WILL BE TOO SOON.

GARY RUDDICK POEMS

ANOTHER LIFETIME YOU WILL BLOOM,

SO MY CHILD DO LET INTO YOUR HEART
SADNESS AND GLOOM,
FOR I FOLLOW AND SEE BY THE LIGHT OF
THE MOON,
HER TWIN IS HER FIRE EVERY BODY SPOKE
A LITTLE TO SOON,
FOR ALL OF US FROM ABOVE HAVE LONG
AGO FLOWN,
 BELIEVE ME MY CHILD YOU ARE NOT
COMING HOME.

THE SYMBOL OF PEACE IS LOVE

THE CROSS IS GUIDED BY THE
HEAVENS ABOVE.

NEVER SHALL YOUR FAITH
FALTER IF IT,

COMES TO PUSH AND SHOVE,

FOR THE FLOWERS AROUND
THESE WORDS,

ARE SENT WITH THE POWER OF
LOVE.

BROUGHT TO YOU THROUGH

THE SOUL OF A DOVE.

CARRIED THRUGH THE SKIES OF HEAVEN

ABOVE.

BROUGHT TO YOU ON THIS DAY

WITH A MESSAGE OF LOVE.

THE VOICE WITHIN!
MANY A CHILD HAS BEEN GIFTED,
IN THEIR MIND MANY A VOICE HAS BEEN SECRETLY WHISPERED,
ONCE IN A WHILE THE VOICE WILL HAVE SHOUTED,
THE CHILDS INSIGHT IN TO THEIR OWN MIND WILL HAVE BECOME CONFUSED AND DOUBTED,
THE SPIRIT INSIDE THE CHILD WILL HAVE BEFORE BIRTH WOULD OF ALREADY OF WOKEN,
FOR INSIDE THE EMBRO OF THE CHILDS MOTHER her voice WILL HAVE CALMLY AND LOVINGLY SPOKEN,
THAT FROM WITHIN WILL HAVE TOLD THE CHILD THAT LOVE IS MUCH MORE THAN A TOKEN,

GARY RUDDICK POEMS

THE CHILDS SPIRIT IS SO STRONG THAT IT COULD NEVER BE BROKEN,
THE VOICE MUST NEVER SPEAK THOSE HURTFUL WORDS OF HATE,
FOR A CHILD MAY UNCONCIUOSLY MAKE A FATAL MISTAKE,
FOR TO THE VOICE THEY DID NOT KNOW HOW TO RELATE,
THE VOICE MAY DECIDE TO USE THE CHILD AS A PIECE OF BAIT,
THE VOICE INSIDE DOES NOT TAKE PRISONERS SOMETIMES THERE ARE NO SURVIVORS, SO PLEASE MY CHILD DO NOT MAKE ANOTHER MISTAKE,
THE DARKNESS WILL SEARCH HIGH AND LOW AND DEATH IS NEVER A DAY TO LATE,
SO LIVE YOUR LIFE DO NOT SIT BACK AND HESITATE,
IVE SEEN MANY A YOUNG CHILD IN A TERRIBLE STATE,
MANY HAVE LOST THEIR LIFELINE DUE TO A DRUG INDUCED STATE,
DEATH WILL BEFALL ALL OF YOU IF YOU LEAVE IT TO LATE,
DEATH HAS NOT OF YET PASSED ITS SELL BY DATE,
ASK YOURSELF IS LIFE A DREAM OR ARE YOU STILL NOT AWAKE,
WHAT WILL YOU DO WHEN IT'S TIME TO TURN THE PAGE AND READ YOUR OWN FATE,

WILL YOUR HEART AND SOUL BE FILLED
WILL LOVE OR WILL YOUR MIND BE FILLED
WITH HATE,
WILL YOU LOOK BACK ON YOUR LIFE AND
WONDER IF TODAY OR TOMORROW HAS
ALREADY PASSESD YOU BY AND IS THE
PRESENT TO LATE,
YOU CAN ALL CHANGE YOUR DESTINY YET
CAN YOU SAVE THE LIFE OF A LOVED ONE
OR YOUR BEST MATE,
FOR IF HIS or her PASSION NOW IS THAT OF A
DRUG INDUCED STATE, IN THIS DAY AND
AGE THERE ARE THOSE THAT YOU CAN NO
LONGER RELATE,
EVEN AN ADULT DOES NOT UNDERSTAND
WHATS IN THEIR BIRTHDAY CAKE,
SO HOW CAN A CHILD UNDERSTAND THE
DRUGS   AND   DRINK   THAT   ARE
COMMERCIALLY THERE FREELY FOR THEM
TO TAKE,
NOW THEIR MINDS ARE NO LONGER IN A
TRANQUIL OR PLACCID STATE,
HOW MUCH LONGER SHALL A PERSON LIE
DOWN AND WAIT,
READING INTO THE LINES AND COLOURS
THAT HAVE BEEN CARVED AND GRAFTED
AND READ INTO TO DECIDE A PERSONS
FATE,
MORE THAN SOME WILL AT SOME STAGE IN
THEIR LIFE WILL HAVE LEARNED HOW TO
EXAGGERATE, THERE ARE THOSE THAT AT

GARY RUDDICK POEMS

TIMES WILL ON THEIR THEORY OF LIFE AS AN INDIVIDUAL OR AS A WHOLE WILL LOOK INTO A MIND AND TRY TO ELABORATE,

THEIR OUR THOSE THAT THROUGH THEIR OWN UNDERSTANDINGS OF LIFE IN THEIR OWN MIND WILL TRY TO FIGURE OUT AND ILLIMINATE,

 THE REASONS WHY A MAN OR A WOMAN HAS GROWN UP TO HATE,

IF THERE IS TIME MANY STORY WILL BE TOLD AND THEY WILL NOT BE USED IN THE TERM OF OUR VOCATION AND THAT IS SOME CHIDREN DO NOT FABRICATE,

MANY A CHILD OR EVEN AN ADULT WILL LEARN TO ADJUST AND IF POSSIBLE HELP OTHERS AND WITH GUIDENCE ONEDAY EDUCATE,

YET THERE IS A TIME AND A PLACE FOR A SPIRITUAL DEBATE,

NO MATTER HOW LONG A CHILD TAKES TIME TO MATURE SOMETIMES IT IS WORTH THE WAIT,

ALL I ASK IS NO MATTER WHAT AILES YOUR CHILD OR ANOTHER BROTHER OR SISTER FATHER OR MOTHERS LOVE

THERE IS NO OTHER JUST PROMISE THOUGH THAT YOU DO NOT LEAVE IT TO LATE,

IF YOU WONDER WHAT ITS LIKE TO HAVE A LOVING AND PHYSICAL PLAYMATE,

JUST BE SURE THAT THEY ARE REALLY AND TRULY ARE YOUR PERFECT SOUL MATE.

Gary Michael Ruddick

Love,xxx.   GARY
MICHAEL RUDDICK

GARY RUDDICK POEMS

THERE ARE NO EXCUSES

Why has man come to hate,
In my mind I can no longer with some relate,
They say they were drunk and it was a stupid mistake,
Yet society does not and never shall except abuse or rape,
Defence council argue, that the child or adult could have made a mistake,
The victim is persecuted and in the witness box begins to cry and shake,
Recalling the moments she layer there frightened her mind was once more about to break,
What dark demon had not for the first time chosen her as just another piece of bait?
In the shadows of the night silently he lay in wait,
Thinking of his next prey he most probably thought that he could not make a mistake,
What system did he use in the silence of his twisted mind or was it just a random date,
Was he induced with drugs that threw out reality that condemned the child to a hysterical state?
Cutting deep into herself she was now filled with hate,
They say time is a healer and that we can only wait,
The next child or woman without special care might not have in her mind that debate,
How can society in money compensate,

When the children do not have a chance to choose their own fate,
Surely it it's down to us to educate,
For if another child were to die would it not be to late,
To simplify my concern I would have to elaborate,
What happened to the innocent young playmate?
In the night all he does is read adult books and fascinate,
When he comes of age he begins to masturbate,
Surely that not how we were meant to educate,
Over time we have reduced ourselves to a malicious state,
Murder drugs crime and rape,
Some countries force you to have a mate,
How many more abused woman and children will it take?
Before society stops being soft and brings back hanging for it wasn't a mistake,
Looking into the past present and future society needs to ratify the mistake,
As it could be your Childs unforeseen fate,
Surely the condemned have chosen their own fate,
Childhood experiences are not how you relate,
Not at the cost at a woman or Childs fate,
For them guilty of such a crime is to terminate,
Another way is to eradicate,
Yet there are those in power, who still think therapy for the abusers take away their hate,
Before they know it their out the prison gate,

GARY RUDDICK POEMS

Another political fucking mistake,
For them that I'm filled with a desire to kill and
hate,

THIS IS MY SANTUARY.

WOULD YOU PLEASE REFRAIN FROM MAKING
TO MUCH NOISE AS LIKE THE YOUNG LADY HAS INDECATED
I COULD VERY WELL BE SLEEPING, SO PLEASE WOULD YOU BE
KIND ENOUGH AS NOT TO DISTURB ME IN THESE RARE AND
PRIECOUS MOMENTS THAT I CAN ESCAPE TO FIND PEACE OF MIND.
IF FOR ANY REASON YOU FEEL THE NEED TO BRING ME BACK
TO CONCIOUSNESS? PLEASE DO NOT AS AT THE MOMENT LIFE IS NOT THAT APPEALING TO ME AT THIS PRECISE MOMENT IN TIME.
IF IT IS THAT IMPORTANT IM, SURE SOMEONE WILL TAKE A MESSAGE.
IF NOONE IS AVAILABLE, YOU MAY PREFER TO COME BACK AT A MORE SUITABLE TIME FOR BOTH OF US.
IM SURE WE CAN MAKE THE EFFORT TO COMPROMISE WITH ONE ANOTHER?
THANK YOU FOR YOUR TIME, ONCE AGAIN MUCH OBLIGED.
SORRY I MISSED YOU THIS TIME, YOU COULD TRY LATER?

GARY RUDDICK POEMS

Gary Michael Ruddick

TO A SECRET CONGREGATION

Life to me has always been a somewhat floored
creation,
Looking back on mankind's evolution,
I have come to the conclusion,
That many a soul is now ready for a mass
expulsion,
Some may state that this is due to mans own
manifestation,
Man has used his own somewhat warped mind to
corrupt every younger generation,
It seems that time has elapsed so fast that this
has become a kind of downward regression,
It seems to me and those of the same congration,
That even a church is no longer a place for a
confession,
Once upon a time the chapel was a place for
meditation,
Now the gardens of those passed away are used
as a sight for excavation,
It comes to mine and the knowledge of those that
are of the same opinion,
That man has exceeded the realms of eternal
redemption,
In my minds eye that is somewhat a kind of a
blessing,
For they are on the verge of reaching extinction,
Self-juvenile regression,
Hate I would not use as a term of expression,

GARY RUDDICK POEMS

It is obvious that mankind has tried to teach or trick those that are empowered with knowledge a lesson,
To others and me that kind of immaturity is somewhat a form of aggression,
What I am seeking is an explanation,
For if they choose to continue with their childish and somewhat stupid expressions,
Then they as in all of mankind shall find that nature has more than one path in the form of a revolution,
Countries are now in the throw of devolution,
Televisions, papers show the aftermath of yet another explosion,
Mothers and their kin no longer look to their fathers for unity and devotion,
War has been declared on many a nation,
Strange how a country would descend on another for the sake of a religion,
Desiring to wipe out a different culture into extinction,
All over some land and a crazy confused population,
Towns and cities bombarded by military government fuelled ammunition,
Families made to suffer just because they represent a different religion,
Or those that feel they are not entitled to live openly in their own jurisdiction,
In this day and age there is no longer any form of communication,

It appears that everything has to be made into
government white paper legislation,
The children of today I feel are no longer being
gilded in the right direction,
Fathers and mothers are worried and they can no
longer live with the stress and the tension,
Screaming and shouting and violence is now a
daily event in many a situation,
Swallowing tablets to help overcome suicidal
thoughts of self-harm and severe depression,
How can society relate to those that do not have
an education?
Does any one these days have an explanation,
Surely the answer is not in chemicals that they
state is a form of medication,
A drug-induced state is not my kind of meditation,
I at least learnt that with my childhood education,
Strange how those that call themselves experts of
the mind, have little knowledge if any at all
concerning the planetary constellation,
For the mind have its own unique patterns of
formulation,
It seems to me that they have misjudged and put
those that now under a government restriction,
Are being forced to take mind-altering medication,
For what they feel is either a delusion or some
kind of dark manifestation,
Yet they are the puppets putting the youth of today
in a state of damnation,
For they are the fraternity that are the spawn of
Satan,

GARY RUDDICK POEMS

Look at the creatures that now walk the earth
once was man now a woman what a fucked up
nation,
So come on doctor where your explanation is,
, In my mind you were long ago forsaken,
You give a seedcase therapy medication,
Yet they have destroyed the trust of any future
generation,
I hold my mind in silence for you all have a
misguided education,
You have ruined lives at the cost of a fabrication,
You state it's not worth the wait so we will lock
them up forever and duration,
Well keep them detained away from civilisation,
As long as we keep them on mind numbing
medication,
Zombiefied is another term of sedation,
We shall take away any form of physical
sensation,
Surely we don't want another revelation,
Strange how some of us had a private education,
Yet that that's something in your report that you
forgot to mention,
You feel that to lock us away and those we will
never be mentioned,
Locked up until were old and unfit psychologically
to deranged to sign for our own pension,
State handouts as a form of compensation,
Yet it's us that teach them about the mind and
give them an education,

For they are to blind to understand what is really going on in the outside world of civilisation,
So they lock those that are of a higher state of consciousness away in all their government backed institutions,
Stating to the public that it is for our own safety and the publics protection,
Strange how they will restrain an individual and force upon them an injection,
They call self-preservation, we are only protecting the next generation, for we don't want this kind of man to have desires   sexual as the opposite sex feel rejection,
So it's not about putting the youth in the right direction,
It's to stop man getting excited over a woman and having an erection,
 This isn't just a place for psychological correction,
It's that their minds have a somewhat floored perfection,
We've read their thoughts and given them every examination,
Yet most are now chronics and they now need long-term rehabilitation,
Us that are doctors we were taught a proper education,
So all I can do is give you an explanation,
Before they come once again and induce another state of sedation,
I'm far too old for retaliation, and I'm too old in the tooth for rehabilitation,

GARY RUDDICK POEMS

Yet I'm here because of false allegations, fitted up by religions and secret organisations,
Spiritually I'm long gone I'm just a figment of your imagination.

TO ALL YOU DADS AND MUMS,
TO ALL YOU DAUGHTERS AND SONS,
TO ALL THE CREATURES THAT LIVE UNDER THE MOON AND THE SUN,
EVEN TO YOU WHO LONG BEFORE WERE THE CHOSEN ONE,
ONEDAY I DREAM THAT LIVE WILL BE FUN,
 BUT FIRST MY FRIENDS WE HAVE TO GET RID OF THE GUNS,
SURELY IT ISNT THAT DIFFCULT TO REVISE YOUR SUMS,
CHIEFS OF THE PAST STOP BEATING YOUR WAR DRUMS,
FOR MOTHERS AND FATHERS ARE LOSING THEIR DAUGHTERS AND SONS,
SO ALL YOU SAILORS AND PIRATES, WHO OF YESTERDAY WHO HAVE DRUNK FROM THE BARREL SWIGGED ON THE RUM,
WHY TODAY DO YOU LOOK SO GLUM,
MUMMIES WITH THEIR BABIES IN THEIR TUM,
DO YOU REMEMBER WHEN YOUR MUMMY USED TO HUMB,
YOU USED TO COMFORT YOURSELF BY SUCKING YOUR THUMB,

EVERY NOW AND THEN YOU GOT A LIGHT
SLAP ON THE BUM,
WONDERING WHERE DID THAT COME FROM,
NOT REALLY UNDERSTANDING WHAT YOU
HAD DONE,
FROM YOUR MOTHER IT NEVER REALLY
STUNG,
I GUESS IT WAS PART OF GROWING UP
THAT'S HALF THE FUN,
 OH TO BE THAT BABY AGAIN GROWING IN
YOU MUM,
YOU KNOW ILL NEVER CHANGE ILL ALWAYS
BE YOUR SON,
FOR I COME FROM INSIDE OF YOU THAT IS
WHERE IM FROM,
IT DOSENT MATTER WHAT WE SAY OR DO, IT
DOSENT MATTER WHAT WEVE DONE,
IT'S WHAT MAKES LIFE SO SPECIAL AND IF I
COULD I WOULD PUT IT IN A SONG,
I REALISE THERE HAVE BEEN TIME WHEN
YOU THINK IVE DONE YOU WRONG,
YET IF I COULD CONFESS MY LOVE FOR YOU
I WOULD PUT IT IN A SONG,
FOR IN MY HEART AND SOUL YOU ALWAYS
WERE THAT BEATIFUL AND ELEGANT SWAN,
FOR ALL OF MY LIFE YOUM HAVE NEVER
DONE ME A WRONG,
I DREAM THAT SPIRITUALLY FROM MY LIFE
YOU SHALL NEVER BE GONE,
FOR YOU ALWAYS WERE THE PEACE MAKER
WITH YOUR MAGIC WAND,

GARY RUDDICK POEMS

THEIR HAS AND NEVER SHALL BE A MORE
LOVING AND TRUSTING FRIEND THAT I AM
MORE FOND,
FROM A SON TO HIS MOTHER I SWEAR TO
KEEP THIS BOND,

TO MOTHER NATURE

TO EVERY GODDESS OF THE SEA, EARTH,
AND SKIES
LOOKING INNOCENTLY INTO THE COLOURS
OF YOUR BEAUTIFUL CRYSTAL CLEAR
HEAVENLY EYES,
I SEARCH INTO YOUR SOUL HOPING THAT I
SHALL ONEDAY ENLIGHTEN YOU WITH THE
COLOURS OF THE RAINBOW AND THE LIGHT
OF THE STARS THE SUN AND THE MOON AND
ALL THE OTHER PLANETS THAT MANKIND
AND WOMANKIND HAS ONLY DREAMED
ABOUT FOR I MY GODDESSES AM AND
ALWAYS SHALL BE FOREVER THE
PERPETUAL OF THE EYES, FOR I HAVE
TRAVELLED THROUGH MANY LIGHT AGES,
SWAM IN THE CLEAREST WARMEST WATERS
WITH THE MERMAIDS GODDESSES OF THE
SEA,
WALKED UPON THE EARTH SINCE THE
BEGINNING OF TIME ON PATHS, ROADS
ACROSS FIELDS SAT IN THE GLADES WITH
THE FAIRY, S MADE DAISY CHAINS WITH

THEM AND FOR THEM, I HAVE WALKED THROUGH THE WILDERNESS WITH THE AMINALS OF MY KINGDOM SHARED A MEAL OR TWO WITH THE LIONS RAN WITH THE CHEETAH, CLIMBED THE TREES WITH THE MONKEYS, THUNDERED THROUGH THE FOREST WITH THE ELEPHANTS SWAM WITH THE DOLPHINS AND THE KILLER WHALES AND GOT BITTEN ONCE OR TWICE BY MY FRIEND THE CRAB, SWAM WITH THE CROCADILE RAN WITH THE RHINO DRANK WITH THE HIPPOPOTAMUS, IVE SHARED A BIT OF CARROT WITH THE HARE AND THE RABBIT AND CHEWED ON A BIT OF WHEAT AND BARLEY WITH MY FIELD MICE,I HAVE FLOWN WITH THE BIRDS OF THE SKIES ALL OVER THE WORLD ,IVE RODE THE HORSE BARE BACK THROUGH THE COUNTRY, IVE FLOWN ON THE DRAGONS BACK AND GLIDED THROUGH THE SUNLIGHT WITH PEGASUS THROUGH THE CLOUDS DARK AND WHITE,I HAVE BEEN GUARDED BY MY BIRDS AND MY DOGS AND COMFORTED BY MY CATS,
MY PATH IS THAT OF THE SKY AND THE LIGHTS SHALL NEVER FADE NO MATTER HOW DARK OR SHADY THOSE THAT HAVE CHOSEN REPRESENT A BOTTOMLESS PIT OF EVIL OF LIES DECEPTION AND DECIET DARKNESS SHALL NOT AND NEVER COULD CLOUD MY SOUL OR TAKE THE LIGHT OUT OF MY SOUL OR THAT OF A CHILD OR AN

GARY RUDDICK POEMS

INNOCENT MAN OR WOMAN I ASK THAT YOU
LIGHT THEIR WAY SO THAT ONEDAY THEY
TO MAY SEE THE COLOUR OF MY LOVE AND
IF YOUR SOUL AND HEART IS AS PURE AND
AS BEAUTIFULLY COLOURED AS MY OWN
AND YOUR EYES ARE THE COLUR OF
MYOWN THEN THE LIGHT SHALL FIND YOU
NOT IN THE COLOUR OF A PERSON BUT IN
THE COLOUR OF THE CLOTH WHICH IS THE
COLOUR OF LOVE THAT OF RELIGION TRUTH
FAITH AND A UNITY THAT WILL BRING FORTH
A PEACE THAT COULD ONEDAY BE
UNIVERSAL, NOT JUST HERE ON EARTH BUT
IN EACH AND EVERY PLANET,ARIES
ATMOSPHERE THROUGH THE MILKY WAY TO
DISTANT GALAXY,S THROUGH THE SOLAR
SYSTEM,S THROUGH THE ASTROLOGICAL
SIGNS OF THE STARS THE PLANETS BIRTH
RIGHT,S AND THE SPIECIESOF EACH ONE OF
THE CREATURES OF THE PLANET EARTH
WHETHER THEY ARE FROM ONE FAMILY
TREE OR ANOTHER WHETHER THEY ARE
FROM A SCHOOL, OF FISH OR THEY HAVE
BEEN BROUGHT UP BY THEIR MOTHER IN
THE NEST EACH AND EVERY CREATURES
TREE WAS IN THE BEGINNING OF TIME
CELESTIAL YET MANKIND HAS CHOSEN WAR
AGAINST ONE ANOTHER AND ON WOMAN
AND CHIDREN SLAUGHTERED THEIR OWN
KIN ,OVER RELIGION THE TONE OF ONES
SKIN ,A PERSONS BELIEFS THEIR FAITH

THEIR PROPERTY THROUGH HATRED AND LOVE HOW DO THEY SLAUGHTER OUT OF LOVE A DUTY TO CARE , TO BE CRUEL TO BE KIND WHAT KIND OF MADNESS IS THAT ,THEY SAY THERE IS METHOD IN MY MADNESS ,YET IN THE REALITY OF MY MIND AT THIS PRECISE MOMENT IN TIME THERE IS NO MADNESS IN MY METHOD.

MY BIRTH SIGN IS THAT OF THE RAM, THE MONTH OF MARCH, THE ARIES, I AM NO LAMB, SO THERE FOR I AM NO SLAUGHTER NIETHER AM I A SLAUGHTERER, OF ANY CREATURE, MY STONE IS THAT OF THE COLOUR AQAUMARINE, MY CONCIEVMENT WAS ON JULY THE FIRST ON MY MOTHERS TWENTY FIRST BIRTHDAY, SO ALL I ASK MOTHER MATURE IS THAT YOU GIVE ME THE KEY TO THE DOOR SO THAT I CAN REGAIN MY FREEDOM AND CONTINUE ON MY OWN DESTINY WHICH IS MY PATH, I HAVE NOT COME HERE TO PREACH THE GOOD BOOK TO YOU NIETHER DO I INTEND TO PREACH TO YOU ABOUT ALL THE OTHER FAITH S OR ARTS THAT MAN AND WOMAN HAVE GOT THEMSELVES INVOLVED IN THEY ARE NOT MY CONCERN FOR THEY HAVE CHOSEN THEIR PATH AND I PRESUME THAT THEIR DESTINY IS NOT THAT OF MINE,MY PATH IS TO TEACH IN A WAY THAT THEY WILL NOT FIND IT THAT EASY TO COMPREHEND MY INTRICATE WAY OF DEALING WITH CERTAIN

GARY RUDDICK POEMS

ISSUES THAT EYE COME FACE TO FACE WITH ON A DAILY BASES, I FOLLOW MY LINE ON MY HAND THAT IS MY DESTINY YET I HAVE TWO HANDS THEY ARE A BOOK OF LIFE MY EYES ARE BRIGHT AND THEY ARE PURPLE,, MY SIGN ARIES, ALSO SPELLS A,SIRE , AND ALSO A,RISE ALSO I,EARS, YET I SHALL LEAVE YOU TO PONDER FOR NOW AND I SHALL REMAIN SILENT AT THE END OF MY PHYSICAL LIFELINE I WILL IN MY SUMMONING UP DECIDE ON LIFE AS A WHOLE THINK AS YOU SEE FIT YET IT IS IRELLEVENT TO MY MIND EYE THAT YOU FEEL THAT I AM NOT IN A POSITION TO MAKE AJUDGEMENT YET MOTHER NATURE IN MY REALITY PHYSICALLY SPIRITUALLY AND MYTHICALLY I AM A GOD FATHER YET I HAVE OTHER RELIGIONS THAT HAVE FAITH IN ME SO IF YOU NEED ENLIGHTENMENT LOOK INTO YOUR MIND BEFORE YOU LOOK INTO MINE FOR I JUST MIGHT BE IN THE DARK AGES BURNING ALL THE RELIGIOUS PAGES OR TURNING THE CARDS OF YOUR PAST PRESENT AND FUTURE CHILDREN OF THE DAY AND NIGHT ,REMEMBER IF YOU PLAY WITH FIREYOU SALL BURN THAT IS A SECRET FROM ONE OF MY BIRDS A GODDESS IN THE SKY.

I SHALL REMAIN SILENT UNTIL THE END OF TIME.

RESPECT

LOVE AND FAITH

YOURS

TRULY

Yours truthfully the universal godfather the lord the Christ the Buddha the wizard love Zeus god of light.

X
X XX
X
GARY

MICHAEL RUDDICK

GARY RUDDICK POEMS

REF. CHURCH OF ENGLAND
NP.600 327B.

22nd August 2004

To whomever this may concern,

Due to the staff shortages and due to management undermining and undercutting the quality of professional and trained personnel resources at Ravenswood House are slowly being pushed out due to management upstairs and those on ground level have decided that due to the government cutting the costs in the public sector those that are incarcerated or detained by the Home Office or those that are placed in the care of their Local Authorities National Health Service (NHS) whether they are a danger to themselves or a danger to the public is not the issue at this precise moment.

What is more important is the care and support that was once given to those detained for whatever reasons are no longer getting the care and support that was at one time available to those that needed to be safe and guarded against themselves or others. Since the NHS introduced the medical fraternity agency, just to undercut one another, the quality of living in the majority of NHS hospitals has somewhat gone down hill.

Communication between nurses and clients has nearly fallen to an all time low. Psychologists and Psychiatrists are far and few between and their presence around the wards are nearly non-existent, except for if those that need their assistance maybe fortunate to gain those allegedly responsible for their well being and their support in re-establishing our return to a safe environment/community. The therapeutic level of nurses has dropped by such a degree of uncertainty not only for the clients here at Ravenswood House but other organisations.

Those that are now being employed by the Government are not of the standards that were once employed by the NHS therefore the quality of care and support that was once given by those that had familiarised themselves in the department of nursing, I feel that their personal statues as professional qualified or untrained nurses has somewhat been undermined by those that supposedly are allegedly stating that we are here to be given a better way of life?

There are now no nurses available to escort those clients into the community for therapeutic or rehabilitation purposes. Therefore the time period in which a client has to be detained is somewhat disturbing not only to the individual but also to the medical team themselves, whether they are discharged into the community by a tribunal or by the hospital management is far too long. I am somewhat troubled by the intake of employees here at Ravenswood House that seem to waltz in day after day without even those that are detained here given as much as a hello and if our behaviour as such or our progress through the services is not to be hindered anymore than necessary. If our attitude is to be documented by those that are aware of certain milestones that we as individuals have had to endure in our development as adults, then I feel, if our personalities are to remain constant throughout our stay here or in any other Government funded establishment would not the whole service (nurses and clients) benefit by returning to the policies that were the structure of the nursing profession and for the benefit of those that have spent years trying to pave a future in nursing what ever level they are deemed capable of achieving.

Budgeting the nurses wages and the funding of the institutions in which I find myself in and unable to get a constant reply from those that unfortunately have to put up with those that are detained indefinitely whether they are employed by the Government or whether we have no choice but to reside here for whatever period of time decided by those that see fit! However, if those of us that are here, I included for the present moment, surely we would be more certain of our position as individuals and our purpose of being detained under the Mental Health Act, no matter how far back it goes into the past.

For I have come to the conclusion that I can no longer learn about myself psychologically, physically and mentally, through medication or therapy and what with the quality of nursing staff dropping to an all time low. I feel that my departure from this establishment is long over due and I feel my departure is imminent in the not to distant horizon because I feel the quality and the input that was once here is no longer available to those that are within the restraints of the sections that have been imposed upon them, by whoever and for whatever reasons. Due to the cost saving that the Government is and has imposed upon all of those in the medical profession. Nobody seems certain if they have enough hours at the end of the calendar month to pay their mortgages let alone repay their student loans or become first time homeowners.

I feel that if the quality of the profession drops, what will that say to the public sector and to the client who finds himself being looked after by someone who is only in the profession for the money and not because they simply care. All I am questioning is whether we, as clients, need another agency as part of a money saving scheme that could jeopardise the whole structure of the health care system for those working within its somewhat stretched limitations.

If the quality of life to rise again, to the level where it was once therapeutic for all involved in the services workforce and clients as a whole, should we not look further a field at those that are in parliament for it is not us that put the government where they are now today and what have they gone and done in return! Undermine and undercut everyone in the service. What a better way to say thank you, what a waste of an education for all parties involved.

Yours Sincerely

Mr. Gary Michael Ruddick.

Gary Michael Ruddick

TRYING TO FIND YOUR FACE IN A CROWD,
DESPARATELY WANTING TO SRCEAM OUT
LOUD,

LONGING TO SEE YOUR FAMILIAR FACE,
LOST AND ALONE IN THIS GOD FORSAKEN
PLACE,

EVERYTIME I SEE YOU MY HEART BEGINS TO
RACE,
IT POUNDS AGAINST MY CHEST WHEN WE
COME FACE TO FACE,

LOOKING AT YOU AS YOU WALK WITH YOUR
AIRS AND GRACE,
ONE MOMENT YOUR THERE THEN YOUR
GONE WITHOUT A TRACE,

LOOKING LOST AND ALONE ONCE AGAIN I
FEEL OUT OF PLACE,
LOOKING FOR THE EXIT I BEGIN TO MAKE
HASTE,

WONDERING IF I SHOULD HAVE GIVEN
CHASE,
YET I DOUBT IF I COULD OF KEPTED UP WITH
YOUR RAPID PACE,

WONDERING IF MY WRITINGS JOIN THE REST
OF THE WASTE,

GARY RUDDICK POEMS

OR ARE THEY IN A FOLDER TIED UP WITH
RIBBON OR LACE,

DO THEY SIT THER IN A FOLDER ON A
WOODEN CASE,
I WISH THEY WERE HIDDEN AWAY IN A
SECRET PLACE,

WILL THEY ONEDAY BE LOST GONE
WITHOUT A TRACE,
THROWN OUT FOR FAR TO LONG HAVE THEY
TAKEN UP WANTED SPACE,

I HOPE MY FEELINGS FOR YOU NO WOMAN
CAN ERASE,
FOR MY LOVE FOR YOU NO WOMAN COULD
REPLACE,

MY LIFE WITHOUT YOU IS NOTHING BUT A
WASTE,
I WONDER IF CUPID HEARS MY PLIGHT AND
FIRES HIS ARROW IN HASTE,

I DREAM ONEDAY THAT WE WILL HOLD
HANDS AND EMBRACE,
WONDERING WHAT YOU WILL WEAR SILK
SATIN OR LACE,

IMAGINING HOW YOUR KISS WILL TASTE,
KNOWING THAT YOU'RE THE PRETTIEST
GIRL IN THE HUMAN RACE,

WONDERING IF TODAY ILL SEE THE SMILE
UPON YOUR FACE,
THINKING OF THE YOUTH IN YOUR EYES I
GET UP AND BEGIN TO PACE,

LOOKING INTO THE MIRROR I LOOK TIRED
AND OUT OF PLACE,
MY MIND IS STRUGGLING TO KEEP AWAKE
YET IKEEP SEEING YOU'RE FACE,
IF I STOP NOW MY THOUGHTS WILL ONLY GO
TO WASTE,
ALL THESE THOUGHTS ILL CARRY WITH ME
TO MY FINAL RESTING PLACE.

Waiting for the curtain to fall.
Hearing the screams deep inside the wall,
Why is it for me that you call?
I don't understand the urgency in your voice,
Why have you made me your first choice?
You stated that you could walk your path alone,
Now you want to return to my home,
Your key shall never unlock my gate,
You have chosen your own fate,
You thought there was a time you thought wrong
for there was no date,
It didn't matter if you lived in a city town or state,
Life and death was never open for a debate,
No one should have died through intercourse with
his or her mate,
How could love so deep have turned to hate,

GARY RUDDICK POEMS

Now it seems we can no longer relate,
What will you say when your stood at heavens gate,
For destiny has already realised your mistake,
Life was always about give and take,
Not about the money you could make,
Under my feet the earth does not shake,
My body or my bones will not break,
It does not alter my path spirits that long ago made my body shake,
For you were only a concoction and your magic was a fake,
It did not matter if I was asleep or I was awake,
Yet there are things that a person must never take,
Your voice was to me a blessing
But to play with my mind and keep me guessing,
That was uncalled for and very distressing,
I guess it was my mind body and soul that you were testing,
Yet why with my life did you start messing?
For I am not the one to go to confession,
One day you shall be taught a lesson,
For it isn't the chemicals that keep me in suppression,
For my lights are in a illuminated formation,
And the stars are not open for a mans expedition,
For life is far older than man-made religion,
The waters will show you your own reflection
yet they could never guide you to place of perfection,

Gary Michael Ruddick

Each and every one of us has our own intuition,
Yet we have to join as one to make a collation,
For if the heavens were to be filled with pollution,
Life would eventually end in extinction,
Every country has its own dereliction,
Yet does it mean that your life is ruled by religion?
For to many years it has caused mayhem and infliction.
Many races have their own inscriptions,
Magazines and papers and all there subscriptions,
Tell of life and all its deceptions,
Yet is there a body to rewrite all the corrections,
This are only my thoughts a sort of reflection,
I guess you could say it's a cross examination,
Talking to you as part of the nation,
I couldn't do it in front of a congregation,
So I speak silently to a new generation,
There are times when you have to use your imagination,
Some people go as far as infiltrating a federation,
That leads to aggravation,
Your beauty and your voice has lead me into a sense of in actuation,
My hopes for you have risen way beyond my imagination,
For one day you may know my truth about the constellation,
Just remember life is down to the mind and the imagination,
Every thought you have has a significant sensation,

GARY RUDDICK POEMS

I cannot as of this moment give you a true explanation,
But in my theories I hope I can give you some insight into my own education,
My mind is not just confused and full of dark manifestations,
For my mind have read at some stage in time the laws and the legislations,
Every person and article has a registration,
That is to further our graduation,
I shall try not to go further a field for you would not understand my comprehension,
And I wouldn't want you to end up on a lost expedition,
Because for you I have very high expectations,
For all I ask from you is that you open your mind and spiritually do a cross examination,
As other wise we just could all end up in damnation,

Gary Michael Ruddick

WHAT WOULD I DO WITHOUT YOU?

WHAT WOULD I DO WITHOUT YOU,
FOR I DO NOT KNOW WHAT I WOULD DO,
I SHALL TELL YOU THAT I AM IN LOVE WITH
YOU,
NO MATTER WHAT YOU SAY OR DO ILL
STAND BY YOU,

IM HERE TODAY FOR THE LOVE OF YOU,
IF ONLY YOU COULD SEE THAT MY LOVE FOR
YOU IS TRUE,
IF ONLY YOU COULD SEE INTO MY SOUL
WHAT I WONDER WOULD YOU DO,
FOR THE COLOURS IN MY EYES ARE PURPLE
AND BLUE,

THERE ISNT ANYTHING THAT I WOULD NOT
DO FOR YOU,
FOR ALL YOU HAVE TO DO IS ASK ME TO,
THAT IS BECAUSE I YEARN TO BE WITH YOU,
YOUR LIGHT SHINES NO MATTER WHAT YOU
DO,

COULD YOUR FEELINGS FOR ME EVER BE
TRUE,
WOULD YOU DO WHAT I ASKED OF YOU,
FOR INTO YOU SOUL I CAN SEE INTO,
AND IN MY HEART I KNOW YOU LOVE ME
TOO,

GARY RUDDICK POEMS

IT DOSENT MATTER WHAT YOU SAY OR DO,
YOUR HEART I WOULD NEVER LEAVE YOU
BLACK AND BLUE,
FOR THAT IS SOMETHING THAT I COULD
NEVER DO,
FOR I HAVE TO MUCH RESPECT FOR YOU,

I ASK MYSAELF MAGICALLY WHAT CAN YOU
DO,
CAN YOU LOVE ME AS MUCH AS I LOVE YOU,
FOR THAT IS WHAT IS WHAT I WISH FOR YOU
TO DO,
BE MINE MY LOVE PLEASE COME TO ME DO,

IF ONLY YOU COULD SEE MY EYES LOOKING
INTO YOU,
WOULD MY SOUL YOU SEE THROUGH,
FOR YOU WOULD KNOW MY HEART
BELONGED TO YOU,
TO WIN YOUR LOVE I NOLONGER KNOW
WHAT IT IS THAT I HAVE TO DO,

I WRITE THIS WITH LOVE FROM ME TO YOU,
FOR THERE IS SOMETHING SERENE IN THE
THINGS THAT YOU DO,
IF ONLY I COULD SPEND THE REST OF MY
LIFE WITH YOU,
FOR I WOULD DO ANYTHING THAT YOU
ASKED ME TOO,

MY LOVE I HAVE ALWAYS BEEN TRUTHFULL
WITH YOU,
FOR I KNOW YOU HAVE BEEN WITH ME TOO,
PLEASE LOVE ME IM BEGGING YOU TOO,
FOR SPIRITUALLY IM COMING OVER TO YOU,

PHYSICALLY I NEED YOU SO DESPARATLY
MY BOO,
MY FEELINGS ARE SO DEEP THAT TO LOSE
YOU I WOULD NOT KNOW WHAT
TO DO,
FOR IN MY DREAMS ALL I WOULD LOVE TO
DO IS SLEEP BESIDE YOU,
PROTECTING YOU ALL THE NIGHT THROUGH.
      WITH LOVE
      GARY
      XXX

GARY RUDDICK POEMS

WHAT'S FOR AFTERS?

DO YOU UNDERSTAND YOUR OWN HAND,
OR DO YOU KILL JUST FOR THE SAKE OF THE
LAND,
DO YOU UNDERSTAND THE SLAUGHTER OF
EVERY LAMB,
BUT WOULD YOU DO IT AT THE PRICE OF A
MAN,

DO YOU UNDERSTAND THE SYMBOL OF THE
FORK,
WHAT WOULD YOU DO IF THE PORK COULD
TALK,
FOR YOU WOULD NOT BE AS ELEGANT AS
THE STORK,
WOULOD YOU STILL BE ABLE TO HOLD YOUR
HEAD UP HIGH AS YOU WALK,

WOULD YOU BE AS DARING AND AS SHARP
AS THE HAWK,
SAT THERE AT THE TABLE WITH YOUR KNIFE
AND FORK,
WONDERING WHAT TODAY THE TRAP
CAUGHT,
STRANGE HOW YOUR FOOD WAS NEVER
BOUGHT,

HOW MANY TIMJES HAVE YOU EATEN THE
COW,

Gary Michael Ruddick

FOR MOST OF YOUR LIFE IT'S BEEN EVERY
WEEK NOW,
DON'T YOU EVER WONDER HOW
VEGETABLES GROW,
DON'T YOU WONDER THAT EVERY THING IS
SO EASY NOW,
HAVE YOU EVER WONDERED HOW THE
BIRDS ARE EASY PICKINGS,
YOU MUST HAVE LOST COUNT OF HOW
MANY SLAUGHTERED CHICKENS,
YOU HAVE HAD COOKING IN YOUR KITCHEN,
WHEN ALL I HEARD WAS RANTING AND
RAVING AND BE WITCHEN,

DO YOU UNDER STAND THE WHALE OR THE
FISH,
IT'S NOT JUST A TASTY OR PRETTY DISH,
IM WRITING THIS FOR A MERMAID, AS THAT'S
MY WISH,
AND IF THE DAY HAD TO COME I WOULD BE
YOUR GIFT,
BUT I WOULD HAVE TO LEAVE YOU AND
RETURN TO THE MIST,
BUT I PROMISE I WOULD NOT LEAVE
WITHOUT GIVING YOU A KISS,
LIFE MY LOVE ALWAYS HAS A TWIST,
MY HAND IS ON MY HEART IN THE FORM OF A
FIST,
THE DAYS ARE TO LONG AND ITS YOU THAT I
MISS,

GARY RUDDICK POEMS

FOR I HOPE THAT YOU ARE A GODDESS AT THE END OF THIS, IF 0NLY WE WERE DOLPHINS WOULDN'T LIFE BE BLISS?
Love
Gary m Ruddick

Gary Michael Ruddick

WHERE IS THE EQUAL EQUALITY?

Do you as a child remember the world was full of
opportunity?
Mum and dad spoke of Open University,
I didn't expect to end up living my life in obscurity,
Looking depressed spending hours looking in the
mi8rror at my self made misery,

Strange how once it's been and gone you can't
change history,
Surely life just can't just be another glorified story,
I sometimes look in the mirror and ignore me,
Don't misunderstand my way of thinking but none
of you are really like me,

I sometimes wonder if you can see inside of me,
I ask myself where is the vision that I used to be,
I ask you is there any hidden quality hidden inside
of you or me,
Are we seriously just a he and a she?

Do we once long ago come from the same tree?
Why did I have to be me why couldn't we stay
together and be as we?
That would have been quite exciting to see,
For I would have given you much more than equal
equality,

If for some reason later in life yours decide that
you cannot follow me,

GARY RUDDICK POEMS

Please I ask that you no longer bother me,
In my minds eye you will always want to care for me,
Sometimes I think you will never let me be.

You shall never learn all of my history,
For there are some things that you are not meant to hear speak or see?
That my friend is why life is more than a mystery,
There are some things in life that are very good quality,

All of us that have must remember losing are virginity,
In the beginning of time that was the first stages of unity,
In my mind the name I had for you was purity,
For you were young fresh and full of innocence and fertility, 29.9.2004

WHIPERING YOUR NAME UNDER MY BREATHE,
HOLDING ONTO YOUR VISION IS NO EASY QUEST,

TO SEE MORE OF YOU IS MORE OF A DESIRE THAN A REQUEST,
HOLDING IN MY BREATH AS I WATCH THE SWELL OF YOUR BREASTS,

Gary Michael Ruddick

I WONDER HOW MANY MORE WAYS WERE
YOU BLESSED,
ONLY YOUR HEART WILL PUT YOUR SOUL TO
THE TEST,

I IMAGINE YOUR HEAD RESTING ON MY
CHEST,
STROKING YOUR HAIR FEELING THE
WARMTH OF YOUR BREATH,

HOLDING ON TO THAT THOUGHT GIVES ME
THE WILL TO CARRY ON,
WATCHING YOU WALK WITH THE SAME
ELIGENCE OF THE FLIGHT OF A SWAN,

WONDERING IF IN YEARS TO COME IF YOULL
STILL REMEMBER MY NAME,
FOR YOU WERE THE ONE THAT KEPT ME
SANE,

KNOWING ONEDAY ILL NEVER SEE YOU
AGAIN,
I KNOW I SHALL HAVE TO FOREVER CARRY
THAT PAIN,

NEVER ON EARTH COULD I LOVE ANOTHER
WOMAN LIKE YOU,
MOST OF ALL IT'S THE LITTLE THINGS THAT
YOU DO,

GARY RUDDICK POEMS

ALL OF MY LIFE IVE LONGED FOR SOMEONE
AS HONEST AS YOU,
NOW YOU'RE HERE I NO LONGER KNOW
WHAT TO DO,

A VERY LONG TIME AGO CUPID CASTE HIS
LOVING ARROW,
IN MY HEART IT HAS BEEN INBEDDED AND
REMOVED ALL MY SORROW,

THE BIRDS SINGING REMIND ME OF YOUR
SOFT VOICE,
MY HEART YEARNS FOR YOU AND I NO
LONGER HAVE A CHOICE,

YOUR BEAUTY IS STILL THAT OF A CHILD,
YOUR MANNER IS THAT OF A WOMAN WHO I
WOULD LOVE TO TURN WILD,

LOOKING DEEPLY INTO YOUR GENTLE
CRYSTAL EYES,
IM REMINDED OF THE CLEAR SUMMER BLUE
SKIES,

I REALISE THAT ONEDAY I SHALL HAVE TO
DRY MY EYES,
KNOWING THAT THIS IS GOING TO BE OUR
LAST GOODBYE,

Why does a child have to return to a tomb?
Why doesn't life continue through the womb?

Where the feeling of love is over to soon,
Surely the earth is more in love with the sun and
the moon,

Maybe a child of nature was born too soon,
Finding his path on his own for he or she was
always well groomed,

Always feeling towards others nothing but love
and a sense of warm,
 Even the bees came to see him in their swarm,

The love of a child will always be torn,
Between man and the and the baby fawn,

The golden field of the corn,
The dazzling lights of the dawn,

The masters of the game with the king and the
pawn,
The ladies presenting them selves on the
immaculate lawn,

The colourful roses with their sharpened thorns,
Presented to the woman whose baby was just
born?

The child awakening with their first yawn,
Unbeknown to the Childs parents the Childs life
spiritually had been sworn,

GARY RUDDICK POEMS

Our lives were mapped out long before we were
born,
Some children grow up top play the role of a king
queen or pawn,

Many a child has passed away not even to see the
mother or father, to whom they were born,
Tears will fall for that is how nature taught us to
mourn,

Lightening and thunder shall always come with the
storm,
Yet the sun will once again rise to bring forth the
warm,

Gary Michael Ruddick

WISHING YOU WAS HERE

Sometimes I feel your presence moving in the air,
There are times when you shine and I know your
there,

At times I wonder if you're my temptress,
Yet you always help me when imp in distress,

So it's you that I should say god bless,
I ask myself are you there as a psychological test,

To you I have nothing deep and dark that I have to
confess,
My friend I no longer feel the need to regress,

For I only end up feeling depressed,
My thoughts to you I have already expressed,

My love for you I could never rest,
For I see into your eyes and I know you are
blessed,

Sometimes with you I am in a bit of a mess,
But your thoughts and feelings I know in my heart
are for the best,

There are moments when with you my heart has
pounded against my chest,
For my want for you is something I try not to
express,

GARY RUDDICK POEMS

There have been times in my life that I cannot
digest,
So I speak with you to help me understand and
express,

If I were to speak with you less,
I think id end up in a right mess,

Sometimes I think I know you less,
But in the long run my friend I know its best,

There are times when I see you with a purple sash
across your chest,
I hope I could one day be your king in the game of
chess,

WONDERING IF I HAVE SEEN YOU BEFORE

LOOKING THROUGH MY WINDOW IN THE
DOOR,
WONDERING IF YOU REALLY UNDERSTOOD
WHAT HAD TAKEN PLACE BEFORE,
LOOKING INTO THE DARKNESS CAGED IN
BEHIND THE CONCRETE WALL,
ASKING MYSELF HAVE I GROWN TO TALL,
LOOKING INTO THE NIGHT SECRETLY ITS
YOU MY LOVE THAT I GENTLY CALL,
SEARCHING OUT YOUR COLOUR IN MY
CRYSTAL BALL,
DATES AND DESTINYS HAVE TO BE
PREDICTED BEFORE THE AUTUMN FALL,
FOR ONCE AGAIN THE WIND SHALL BLOW
AND THE LEAVES SHALL FALL,
CAGED FACES LOOKING OUT FROM THE
PRISON WALLS,
WONDERING IF THEY SHOULD WAIT UNTIL
THAT LETTER OR A SECRET MESSAGE IN
THE PHONE CALL,
LISTENING ALL THROUGH THE NIGHT FOR
THE EARLY MAGPIES CALL,
OTHERS NOT SO FORTUNATE WILL HEAR
THE SCREECH OF THE RAVENS CALL,
MANY A SOUL HAVE TAKEN FLIGHT INTO THE
ABYSS THEY BEGIN TO FALL,
FOR IT WAS NOT THE RAVENS SHRILL ALAS
IT WAS ITS MASTERS CALL,

GARY RUDDICK POEMS

LONG AGO THEY TRIED TO TAKE HIM FOR A FOOL,
COVER HIS EYES WITH DYED BLACK WOOL,
LITTLE DID THEY KNOW HE DELUDED THEM AND HE KEPTED HIS COOL,
IN THE DARKNESS HE ALWAYS HAD HIS MAGICAL GIFT THAT HE USED AS HIS ONLY TOOL,
HE LEARNED THROUGH YEARS OF LISTENING TO THE SPIECES OF THE WORLD YET HE ALWAYS HAD HIS OWN PROTOCAL,
BOOKS OF KNOWLEDGE AND WISDOM IN HIS MIND WERE ONLY FOR A FOOL,
PICTURES HE COULD UNDERSTAND ONLY THOSE OF GODS AND GODDESSES SPOKE TO HIM THROUGH THEIR DRESS AND THEIR POSTURE HE DREAMED ONEDAY THEY WOULD RULE,
ONLY IF THEY LISTENED TO HIS WISDOM YET THEY HAD TO KEEP THEIR COOL,
FOR MANKIND HAD TAKEN HIM FOR A FOOL,
FOR HE WAS NOT A LAMB TO THE SLAUGTER AS THEY HAD TRIED THAT SACRIFICE BEFORE,
THIS TIME THOUGH IT WAS NATURES CALL,
THEY TRIED TO SLAUGHTER HIM INSIDE THE PRISON WALL,
BUT A BIRD OF PREY HELPED HIM OVER THE WALL,
FOR ALL OF LIFE WOULD CEASE THE HEAVENS ABOVE WOULD FALL,

Gary Michael Ruddick

ALONG TIME AGO ON A HORNED TUSK
SILENTLY HE DID CALL,
A WOMAN TRIED TO WARN HIM YET HE GAVE
HER ACCESS INTO HIS CASTLE BEHIND HIS
DEFENSIVE WALL,
NOW HE HAS RETURNED TO NATURE AS
THEY TOOK HIM FOR A FOOL

Wondering if you'll ever fight for a cause,
Trying to regain your freedom locked inside a
room of just bricks and doors,

Inside your mind you're fighting a silent war,
Feeling frightened something, which you've never
felt before,

Not knowing anymore what's wrong or right,
No window to guide you through the day and
night,

You can no longer tell the difference between
black and white,
All you've ever wanted was to stand there and
fight,

Condemned before you could even walk,
Struck down as soon as you could talk,

Feeling in you began to develop that you didn't
understand,

GARY RUDDICK POEMS

No one offered you guidance or a helping hand,

They took away your liberty right then you knew
you were damned,
They told you that your life was never planned,

You never learned to read or write something you
were never taught,
No one even gave you a chance or even a second
thought,

Before you were born you were discussed in
another statistic report,
They thought it best if your mother were to abort,

They even took it through the high court,
Yet you won the love and the public support,

You have now reached a mature age,
Yet you look through mindless sunken eyes lost in
a daze,

You try to recall that the drugs were just a phase,
Your mind tries to remember but you're lost in a
haze,

What will be written on the coroner's final page?
Life to him was a play and he died on stage,

He should have been aborted for his mum was
under age,

Gary Michael Ruddick

His father he never knew died in a prison cage,

GARY RUDDICK POEMS

WORD ASSOCIATION

Do you ever look into the mirror at your own reflection?
Looking for lines, wishing that the ageing process would miraculously reverse in the opposite direction,
Girls I know makeup is not really much of compensation,
Yet your maturity and beauty give me the strength and I hope the wisdom,
To unite you with the heavens that be and it is your love and sincerity and your dreams of tranquillity for you of the fairer sex are my inspiration,
To unite the world as one may it be through race religion or culture holistically and spiritually realistically not mythically whether it be emotionally,
Man has to respect a woman honourably treat her as an equal respectfully,
Not just for the moment but also continuously for eternity for a woman's love and trust is more than heavenly,
I do not understand how a man could even contemplate killing a woman or their kin murderously,
And I do not understand for the life of me how a man could even consider molesting a child or a woman for those thoughts could never enter my mind honestly,

For my thought process does not and never could nor would enter such brutality,
For that is some kind of perverse abnormality,
The depths of man depravity not all man a percentage has lost their sanity,
To me it seems that those that have crossed the boundaries of normality,
Should not return to the light spiritually, for eternity,
For they have committed the sacred vowels of humanity spiritually,
I do not understand the thinking of those in government positions, who deem them fit for society,
How can a woman and her child be safe in the community?
When the government protects those guilty of perversity with anonymity,
I feel as a father that the judicial system has made a mockery out of society,
As the days pass by I feel the light slowly fade from my soul for it is not I that has lost their sanity,
This place to me is not my reality neither is my sanctuary,
And it could never be a place that heaven calls purgatory,
If death should ever come before me all I ask is that you read my story.

YOU ARE MY GUESTS

GARY RUDDICK POEMS

Life has more than just one path for every tree has its own crest,
Many a creature have laid an egg in their family nest,
Any creature born from this earth it is you and your children that I invest,
For it has come to my attention that mankind has put the heavens to the test,

There are those that mock and those that laugh at those unfortunate to not of been blest,
Isn't it time that all religions in the past and present and I hope the not too distant future came to gather as one and put a child and their parents mind at rest,
I shall see in my lifetime if those that truly know me think that once I am laid to rest,
That what I write in these scripts has been wrote in not jest,

As I see with my senses the planets are in turmoil and dangerously close to civil unrest, it seems to me that each nation has an armed force that have regressed,
Communities around the globe whether they are religious or whatever nationalities they are from brotherhoods have become stressed,
Fighting and killing on e another over faiths surely this is not the way forward this is not progress,

If you s that are in power surely you are intelligent
and wise enough to debate over your beliefs
whether they be held in congress,
Or if you choose to enter a holy house, the stature
of the priest or priestess,
They too are there only as a guest,
The world knows, it seems, is in a spiritual
process,
Of losing the path of light for many a child has
been born and passed away without even the
thought of being blessed,
Myself it concerns me for I am troubled dismayed
and depressed,
Yet how do you open your heart and your soul for
I am not here for you to confess?
Yet there are those that look at me with a smile of
surprise for it you that have yet to pass the
spiritual test,
Show me something that would make me
impressed,
For I do not need an invitation as a patient client
or any form of guest,
For on my hand I have a sacred spiritual crest,
If I were to choose to venture on a holy quest,
I would only allow those innocent and pure to join
me as my guests,
Yet could your souls truly understand my mind
read between the lines and be able to digest,
That this is not some far-fetched idealistic scheme
that has in my mind has just begun to manifest,

GARY RUDDICK POEMS

This is not about power or might or who is the smartest or what country are the best,
It's a universal obligation to those that have died for freedom honour and love to ease those that are still suffering and dying for a cause for stopping the unrest,
For fighting is not my way of a peaceful conquest,
For there comes a time in a persons life when they lay down their arms and decide morally and spiritually to become a pacifist
Every man and woman has the sense to realise that their has to come a time where every religion and country has to lay down their arms for as children each one of you are heavenly blessed,
The time shall one day arrive for my mind and body to lie down and forever be put to rest,
My spirit shall guide those as it always has done since the light evolved from Mother Nature's nest,
As long as the blood runs through her veins as Mother Nature is your earth with my hand upon my chest,
Maybe next time if the heavens permit I may be nurtured from your breast,
I only pray that you would want me in your heart and soul as your GUEST,
For in my eyes you are more than a guide for you are a heavenly lovely goddess,
I pray and I hope with love and faith, god bless,
Love
GARY
XXX

Gary Michael Ruddick

You are my light.
When you appear in the glorious daylight,
In my heart it is love at first sight,
If I were to see you silhouette in the moonlight,
I would know that my feelings for you were right,
The candle that I hold for you shall always burn into the night,
Showing you a path that even the blind can see the light
My love my spirit since we first meet has been lifted into the light,
For you I would open up the heavens and show you the path into the twilight,
Showing you the path that for you they hold your spirit for you are my guiding light,
All my life I have been on a magical,
Plight, Alone on the skyline watching your presence as you sleep peacefully into the night,
Hoping and praying that your path was not just on the right,
Looking into your soul all I see is the sunlight,
I have fallen in love with you and I could not put up a struggle or even have the strength to fight,
If I were to gently kiss you would it be right,
Would you turn on me with all your might?
Would then again you show my the way into the light,
Or would you lock my path away into the night,
I dream wishfully that one-day you will ask me to hold you tight,

GARY RUDDICK POEMS

Guiding me out of the dark into the your light,
Where together we could put the world to rights,
Love Gary xxxxxxxxxxxxx

YOU COULD HAVE THOUGHT

It was never about the money to the churches you
brought,
For to give was what you have always been
taught,

To give would always lighten your soul,
It was never about what I had stole,

If you look at life as a whole,
Not at the individual for that would cause turmoil,

Look at the earth and not at the soul,
Look at the young and not just the old,

People have and still are being sold
I presume one day our sins will eventually take
there toll,

Ell we be left in the open to shiver alone in the
cold,
Will your anger break you and will you explode,

Will your skin grow grey your beauty corrode,
Could you ever shed your heavy load?

Some speeches are never in the open to be
spoken,
For wars are created at the press of a button,

GARY RUDDICK POEMS

Punishment was never meant to come in the form of the hanged,
For that's putting you amongst the damned,

If you're a victim of a pointless death,
Come back to life its more than an invitation it's like a request,

Put your faith to the test,
Life was never meant to a test,

It isn't about the next conquest,
Welcome to the world for you are more than a guest, god bless.

The
Emblem
Of Peace
Is Love

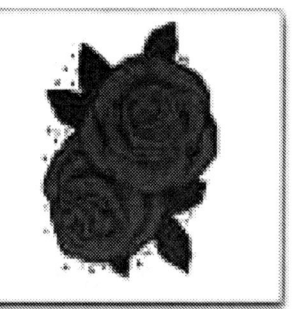

THE SYMBOL OF PEACE IS LOVE

Gary Michael Ruddick

THE CROSS IS GUIDED BY THE HEAVENS ABOVE.

NEVER SHALL YOUR FAITH FALTER IF IT,

COMES TO PUSH AND SHOVE,

FOR THE FLOWERS AROUND THESE WORDS,

ARE SENT WITH THE POWER OF LOVE.

BROUGHT TO YOU THROUGH

THE SOUL OF A DOVE.

CARRIED THRUGH THE SKIES OF HEAVEN

ABOVE.

BROUGHT TO YOU ON THIS DAY

WITH A MESSAGE OF LOVE.

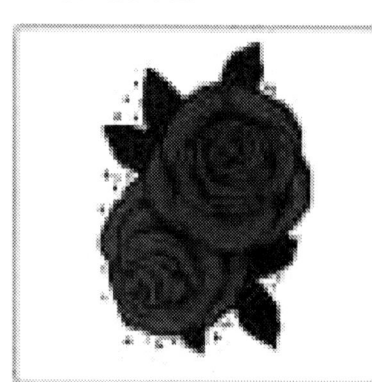

Lightning Source UK Ltd.
Milton Keynes UK
26 January 2010
149098UK00001BB/1/A